THE COMPLETE DIABETES COOKBOOK

More than 500 Simple and Easy Recipes for Balanced
Meals and Healthy Living

Lory Crocker

THE COMPLETE
DIABETES
COOKBOOK

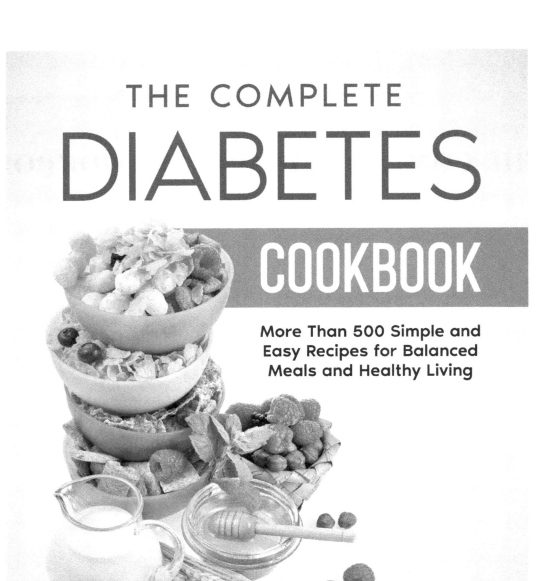

More Than 500 Simple and Easy Recipes for Balanced Meals and Healthy Living

Lory Crocker

Table of Contents

DIABETIC DATE DAINTIES

2 eggs
1 1/2 tsp. liquid sweetener
1 1/2 tsp. baking powder
1/3 c. dates, chopped
1/4 c. flour
1/2 c. nuts
1 1/2 c. bread crumbs

Beat eggs, sweetener and baking powder. Add dates, flour and nuts. Stir in bread crumbs. Chill, then measure by teaspoon on a greased cookie sheet. Bake at 375 degrees for 12 minutes.

SUGAR - FREE CRANBERRY RELISH

2 c. cranberries
2 apples
1 c. orange juice

Grind together the cranberries and apples, using a sweet apple. (May also use blender). Add orange juice, chopped nuts and sweetener to taste. Refrigerate several hours before using.

IT COULD BE A SNICKERS BAR

12 oz. soft diet ice cream
1 c. diet Cool Whip
1/4 c. chunky peanut butter
1 pkg. sugar-free butterscotch pudding (dry)
3 oz. Grape-Nuts cereal

Mix first 4 ingredients in mixer, then stir in cereal. Pour into 8 inch square pan. Cover and freeze. Makes 4 servings.

BAKED CHICKEN FOR ONE

1 (3 oz.) chicken breast, boned & skinned
2 tbsp. (any brand) bottled diet Italian dressing

Marinate chicken in dressing overnight in covered casserole. Bake for one hour at 350 degrees. No additional seasonings are necessary. Will be very tender and juicy,.

CHOCOLATE CHIP COOKIES

1/4 c. margarine
1 tbsp. granulated fructose
1 egg
1 tsp. vanilla extract
3/4 c. flour
1/4 tsp. salt
1/2 c. mini semi-sweet chocolate chips

Cream together margarine and fructose, beat in egg, water and vanilla. Combine flour, baking soda and salt in sifter. Sift dry ingredients into creamed mixture, stirring to blend thoroughly. Stir in chocolate chips. Drop by teaspoonsful onto lightly greased cookie sheet about 2 inches apart. Bake at 375 degrees for 8 to 10 minutes. Makes 30 cookies.

ORANGE RICE

1 c. rice, uncooked
1 c. water
1 c. orange juice
1 tsp. reduced calorie margarine
Dash of salt
1 tbsp. orange rind, freshly grated
1/2 c. fresh orange sections, seeded

In a 2-quart microwave safe casserole, combine the rice, water, orange juice, margarine and salt. Cover, microwave on High for 5 minutes. Stir in the orange rind. Turn the bowl 1/4 turn. Microwave on High for an additional 10 minutes, turning the bowl after 5 minutes. Do not uncover the bowl. Allow to set covered for an additional 10 minutes or until all of the liquids have been absorbed. Immediately before serving, fluff with a fork, add orange sections and mix gently. Serve with pride. Makes about 6 (100 calories) servings.

BLACK BOTTOM PIE

--GRAHAM CRACKER CRUST:--

1 1/4 c. graham cracker crumbs
1/2 c. diet margarine

--FILLING--

1 envelope unflavored gelatin
3/4 c. part-skim ricotta cheese
12 packets sweetener
1 packet low-calorie whipped topping mix
1 1/2 c. skim milk
1 tbsp. vanilla extract
1/4 c. cocoa

Combine crumbs with diet margarine by cutting in softened margarine until mixture resembles coarse crumbs. Press firmly in bottom and sides of 8 or 9 inch pie pan. Bake in preheated 350 degree oven for 8 to 10 minutes. Cool. In small saucepan, sprinkle gelatin over 1/2 cup skim milk. Let stand one minute.

Heat, stirring constantly until gelatin dissolves. In blender or food processor, blend ricotta until smooth and add gelatin mixture, remaining 1 cup milk and vanilla. Continue blending until completely smooth. Remove half the mixture, set aside. To mixture still in blender, add 6 packs sugar substitute and cocoa. Blend thoroughly. Pour blender mixture into crust, chill for 30 minutes or until partially set. At the same time, chill remaining mixture for 30 minutes.

Prepare whipped topping mix according to package directions gradually adding remaining 6 packets sugar substitute. Whisk into reserved, chilled mixture until blended smoothly. Spoon over chocolate layer; chill until set. Garnish with dusting of cocoa. Makes one (8 or 9 inch) pie or 8 servings.

CHICKEN BREASTS WITH CARROT AND ZUCCHINI STUFFING

2 small (whole) skinless, boneless chicken breasts
1 c. carrots, shredded (about 2 sm.)
1 c. zucchini, shredded (about 1 med.)
1 tsp. salt
1/4 tsp. poultry seasoning
1 envelope chicken-flavored bouillon
1/4 c. water

In medium bowl, combine carrots, zucchini, salt and poultry seasoning. Spoon about 1/2 cup mixture into each pocket (each breast should open similar to a butterfly); secure with toothpicks. In place chicken in a Med size skillet, sprinkle with bouillon.

Add water to skillet and cook over medium high heat, heat to boiling. Reduce heat to low; cover and simmer about 40 minutes or until chicken is fork tender. Remove toothpicks. Makes 4 servings, 180 calories per serving.

SUGARLESS CAKE

1 c. dates, chopped
1 c. prunes, chopped
1 c. raisins
1 c. cold water
1 stick margarine, melted
2 eggs
1 tsp. baking soda
1/4 tsp. salt
1 c. plain flour
1 c. nuts, chopped
1/4 tsp. cinnamon
1/4 tsp. nutmeg
1 tsp. vanilla

Boil dates and prunes in the one cup of water for 3 minutes; add margarine and raisins and let cool. Mix flour, soda, salt, eggs, nuts, spices and vanilla. Add to fruit mixture. Stir to blend. Pour into baking dish. Bake at 350 degrees for 25 to 30 minutes.

DIABETIC ORANGE SUNBEAMS

1 1/2 c. all-purpose flour
1 tsp. baking powder
1/4 tsp. salt
1/2 c. shortening
1/2 c. raisins
1 egg
2 tbsp. orange juice
2 tsp. grated orange rind
1 1/2 tsp. Sucaryl

Sift together flour, baking powder and salt. Cut in shortening until crumbly. Add all at once: raisins, eggs, orange juice, orange rind and Sucaryl. Mix well. Make into small balls; flatten on cookie sheet. Bake 12 to 15 minutes at 375 degrees.

ALMOND BISCUIT RING

1/4 c. granulated brown sugar, replacement
2 tbsp. diatetic maple syrup
2 tsp. reduced calorie margarine
2 tsp. water
1/3 c. almonds, coarsely chopped
1 (8 oz.) tube refrigerator biscuits

In a 1 1/2 quart microwave safe casserole, combine the brown sugar replacement, maple syrup, margarine and water. Cover with a paper towel and microwave on high for one minute. Allow to sit, covered for one minute, then stir to mix in the melted margarine. Stir in the almonds. Cut each of the biscuits into four pieces.

Roll each piece into a ball. Dip each piece into the syrup mixture then place in a microwave safe ring mold. Arrange all coated balls uniformly around the ring mold. Pour any remaining syrup over the balls in the mold.

Microwave on medium (50% power) for 5 to 6 minutes, turning the mold 1/4 turn after each two minutes. Remove from oven and immediately cover with waxed paper. Allow to sit undisturbed 5 minutes; then turn out onto a serving dish. Divide into 10 servings. About 80 calories per serving.

BANANA SPLIT PIE

1 graham cracker crust
1 (4 oz.) pkg. sugar-free instant vanilla pudding mix
2 c. low-fat milk
2 bananas, sliced
1 (15 oz.) can crushed pineapple
1 c. Cool Whip
1 tsp. vanilla
1/2 c. pecans, chopped

Mix pudding with milk and beat until thick, pour into crust. Put bananas over pudding. Squeeze pineapple to remove all juice. Sprinkle on top of bananas. Cover with Cool Whip, sprinkle pecans on top. Chill well.

FRUIT DIP

1 c. plain yogurt
8 oz. light cream
8 packets Equal sugar
1 tsp. vanilla.

 Mix all ingredients together.

BROWNIE TORTE

1 1/2 c. chilled whipping cream
3 tbsp. Fruit Sweet or to taste
1 tsp. vanilla

Prepare Fudge Sweet Brownies (see recipe below). Whip cream, Fruit Sweet and vanilla and use as filling and topping for layers of brownies. Low-Fat Substitute: About 3 cups frozen whipped topping, thawed. Substitute your favorite flavoring for the vanilla, such as 1 tablespoon instant coffee or 1 tablespoon concentrated orange juice.

FUDGE SWEET BROWNIES

2/3 c. flour
1/2 tsp. baking powder
2 eggs, beaten well
1/2 c. melted butter or oil
1/2 c. Fudge Sweet, softened
1/2 c. Fruit Sweet
1 tsp. vanilla
1/2 c. walnuts, chopped

Sift flour and baking powder; set aside. Blend the eggs, butter or oil, Fudge Sweet, Fruit Sweet and vanilla. Add the flour mixture and blend thoroughly. Add walnuts. Pour mixture into greased and floured 8"x8" baking pan. Bake at 350 degrees for about 15 minutes, until cake springs back at a light touch. Doubled recipe will fit into double size cookie pan.

FROZEN APRICOT MOUSSE

1 c. apricot apple butter
1/2 c. whipping cream
2 egg whites
2 tbsp. Fruit Sweet

Beat egg whites until stiff but not dry. Fold into the apricot apple butter. Whip the cream until stiff, adding the Fruit Sweet. Fold the whipped cream into the apricot mixture. Freeze.

FRUIT LEATHER

Place a sheet of plastic wrap in the bottom of a cookie sheet. Smooth a thin layer of fruit butter with the edge of a pancake turner. Place in the oven to dry at the lowest heat, about 120, for about 2 hours, or until dry, then remove and cool. Peel off and roll in plastic wrap. For variety, sprinkle with finely chopped walnuts before drying.

FRUIT SALAD TOPPING

1 1/2 c. milk (skim or 1%)
1 (3 oz.) sugar free vanilla pudding

Add: 2 tbsp. frozen orange juice concentrate
1 tsp. grated orange peel (opt.)

Can be served as a side dish with mixed fruit (fresh) or mix fruit and topping in bowl.

RASPBERRY MOUSSE

2/3 c. Strawberry Fanciful
1/8 tsp. cream of tartar
2 egg whites
1/2 c. whipping cream

Add cream of tartar to egg whites, beat until stiff, but not dry. Fold into Strawberry Fanciful. Fold the whipped cream into the fruit mixture. Chill before serving or freeze for frozen mousse. For flavor variation try: Strawberry, blueberry, orange pineapple, pineapple berry or peach.

GOLDEN CARROT PIE

2 eggs
1/4 tsp. ground cinnamon
Pinch salt
1/2 c. Fruit Sweet
9" pie shell
Dash ground nutmeg
1/8 tsp. ground ginger
1 c. cooked carrots, riced or mashed
1/2 c. heavy cream

Beat the eggs, nutmeg, cinnamon, ginger and salt until thoroughly blended. Add the carrots and stir well. Pour in the Fruit Sweet and cream and stir until completely blended. Pour the filling into the pie shell and bake at 350 degrees for 35 minutes or until a knife inserted in the center comes clean. Serve with whipped topping.

APPLESAUCE CAKE

2 eggs, well beaten
1 c. Apple Butter
1 1/2 c. flour
1/2 c. raisins
1/2 c. butter, melted
1/2 c. Fruit Sweet
1 1/2 tsp. baking soda
1/2 c. chopped walnuts

Combine the eggs, butter and apple butter. Sift the flour and bake soda. Add the walnuts and raisins to the flour mixture and blend. Add the flour mixture to the egg mixture alternately with the Fruit Sweet. Pour the batter into a greased tube pan and bake at 375 degrees for 30 to 35 minutes. Turn out and cool before serving. Serve with whipped cream.

EASY CHOCOLATE GRAHAM TORTE

Line 13"x9"x2" pan with a layer of graham cracker squares. Prepare 1 large (6 oz.) package of instant sugar-free chocolate pudding as directed on the package. Spread over graham cracker layer. Place in refrigerator to let set a little.

Layer another layer of graham cracker squares over the pudding. Prepare a second package of chocolate pudding as above and spread over graham crackers. *Refrigerate.* Torte may be topped with whipped cream or Dream Whip when served. This easy dessert is one that diabetics may enjoy.

FANCIFUL FREEZE

4 ripe bananas, peeled
1/2 c. Raspberry Fanciful

Wrap bananas in plastic wrap and freeze overnight. Remove from freezer, break into 4 or 5 pieces and let stand at room temperature for about 10 minutes to slightly soften for the processor.   Blend the bananas in a processor or blender until creamy. Add the Raspberry (or other flavor) Fanciful and blend briefly. This can be served immediately, or stored in the freezer. Serves 4.

NO-SUGAR CUSTARD

6 egg yolks
1/4 c. Fruit Sweet
1/2 c. flour
2 c. milk
1 tsp. vanilla
1 tbsp. butter

In a medium bowl, beat egg yolks and Fruit Sweet until thick and pale. While continuing to beat, gradually sift in flour. Pour into a saucepan and place over low heat on the stove and gradually add milk and vanilla. Cook, stirring constantly, until mixture has thickened to a custard consistency, about 15 minutes. Remove from heat. Melt butter and pour over custard to prevent a skin from forming while it cools. Makes 3 cups.

CHOCOLATE CAKE

2 eggs, beaten
1/2 c. butter, melted
1 c. strawberry apple butter
1 tsp. vanilla
5 tbsp. milk
3/4 c. Fudge Sweet Topping
5 tbsp. Fruit Sweet

2 c. flour
2 tsp. baking powder

Combine eggs, butter, strawberry apple butter and vanilla. Place the covered jar of Fudge Sweet into hot water to thin. Add the milk, Fudge Sweet and Fruit Sweet to the butter mixture. Sift the flour and baking soda together and blend with the wet mixture.   Pour into two greased and floured 9" round tins or equivalent. Bake at 350 degrees for 40 minutes. Cool. Top with whipped cream.

ORANGE MINCE CAKE

2 eggs, well beaten
1/3 c. Fruit Sweet
1 1/2 c. flour
1 1/2 tsp. baking powder
1/4 c. butter
1 c. Fruit Mincemeat
1 tsp. baking soda

Beat eggs, melt butter and add to Mincemeat and Fruit Sweet. Sift dry ingredients, add to mincemeat mix and blend. Spoon and smooth batter into oiled and floured 8" baking pan. Bake at 350 degrees for approximately 25 minutes. Top with Orange Cream Cheese Topping.
--ORANGE CREAM CHEESE FROSTING--

6 oz. cream cheese
2 tbsp. Fruit Sweet
2 tbsp. concentrated orange juice

 Blend all ingredients together. Use on Orange Mince Cake.

LO-CAL CHEESE CAKE

12 oz. low fat Ricotta cheese
4 eggs, separated
3/4 c. Fruit Sweet
Grated peel of 1 lemon
3 graham crackers, finely crushed

12 oz. low fat cottage cheese
2/3 c. non-instant milk powder
5 tbsp. lemon juice or to taste
2 tsp. pure vanilla
Butter or oleo for pan

Put cheese in process with egg yolks and Fruit Sweet and blend. Add milk, powder and process until smooth. Add vanilla, lemon juice and peel to cheese mixture. Blend until smooth. Beat egg whites until frothy, then add to the processor and blend for about 2 seconds, until mixed. Butter the bottom and 1/2 way up the sides of a 9" springform pan.

Pour the graham cracker crumbs into the pan and shake until buttered area is coated. Leave any extra on the bottom. Pour cheesecake mixture into pan and bake at 350 degrees with a pan of water in the oven to prevent drying.   Bake for 45 minutes or until inserted knife emerges clean. Cool. May serve with Wax Orchards All-Fruit Fanciful preserve of your choice. *Variations: All cottage or all ricotta cheese may be used. For standard cream cheese cake, substitute 24 ounces cream cheese, 3 eggs, 1/2 cup powdered milk and 2/3 cup Fruit Sweet. Adjust lemon.*

APRICOT PINEAPPLE CAKE

2 eggs, beaten
3/4 c. Apricot Apple Butter
1/2 c. dried apricots, chopped fine
2 tsp. baking soda
1/2 c. butter, melted
1/2 c. drained, crushed pineapple
2 c. flour
1/2 c. Fruit Sweet

Combine the eggs, butter, Apricot Apple Butter, pineapple and dried apricots until thoroughly blended. Mix the flour and baking soda together, then combine with the egg mixture alternately with the Fruit Sweet. Mix until the batter is smooth. Bake in a 9"x12" greased and floured pan at 340 degrees for 40 minutes or until cake springs back when pressed lightly. Remove the cake from the oven. Cool, turn out and cool completely. Flavor is usually better the next day.

REFRIGERATOR BRAN MUFFINS

1 1/2 c. apple juice
1 c. butter, melted
4 well beaten eggs
4 c. buttermilk
5 tsp. baking soda
2 c. processed Bran Buds
1 c. Fruit Sweet
4 c. ready-to-eat bran cereal
5 c. flour
1 tsp. salt

Pour the juice into a medium saucepan and bring to a boil over high heat. Remove, pour in the Bran Buds and stir well. Let the mixture stand for several minutes. Combine the butter, Fruit Sweet and eggs and beat well. Then stir in the bran cereal. Pour in the buttermilk and stir well, then add the flour, baking soda and salt. Beat the batter until it is thoroughly blended.

Add the juice and Bran Buds and stir the batter until well blended. Drop several teaspoonfuls of batter into each greased muffin cup. Bake at 400 degrees for 15 minutes or until the center of each muffin is done. The batter can be stored in the refrigerator for up to 6 weeks and used as needed. Fruit and nuts, such as raisins, cranberries, bananas and walnuts, can be finely chopped, tossed with a little flour can also be used to add a little variety.

BUTTER POUNDCAKE

2 eggs, separated
6 tbsp. butter, softened
2 tsp. vanilla
2 tsp. baking powder
4 tbsp. whipping cream
3/4 c. Fruit Sweet
1 3/4 c. sifted cake flour
1 tsp. baking soda

Beat the egg yolks well. Add cream, butter, Fruit Sweet and vanilla and beat to blend well. Set aside. Sift the flour, baking powder and baking soda together and set aside in a small bowl. In a medium size bowl, slowly blend the flour mixture and the liquid mixture in small amounts at a time until well mixed. Beat until smooth.

In a separate bowl, beat egg whites until stiff but not dry. Stir a third of the whites into the batter and then gently fold in the remainder. Spoon into a greased and floured 9" pan. Bake in a preheated 350 degree oven for 25 to 35 minutes or until an inserted straw or toothpick comes out dry. Cool for about 5 minutes before turning out onto rack.

TORTE AU CHOCOLA

1 3/4 c. cake flour, sifted
1/43 tsp. salt
3 tsp. baking powder
1/2 tsp. cinnamon
4 eggs, separated
1/2 c. melted butter or oil
3/4 c. Fruit Sweet
3/4 c. Fudge Sweet
1 tsp. vanilla
1/2 c. milk

Sift dry ingredients together and set aside. Combine the butter or oil, Fruit Sweet, Fudge Sweet and vanilla. Add the yolks to the liquid mixture, blending one at a time. Add the flour mixture to the liquid mixture alternately with the milk. Whip the egg whites to stiff peaks and fold in gently but thoroughly. Bake at 350 degrees for 1/2 hour in 2 (9") round greased and floured tins. Test. Cake will spring back when lightly touched. *For a drier cake, bake until the cake draws away from the edge of the pan*. Cool.
--FILLING--

1 (8 oz.) pkg. cream cheese
3 tbsp. Fruit Sweet
1 tsp. vanilla

Blend together. Cream cheese may be warmed slightly to soften for blending. Fill cake, then frost with whipped cream sweetened to taste with Fruit Sweet, flavored with vanilla or your favorite flavoring.

Drizzle melted Fruit Sweet around edge of cake. *optional - put thinly sliced strawberries on top.*

DIABETIC OATMEAL PEANUT BUTTER COOKIES

2/3 c. oatmeal
2 c. flour
1 tsp. lite salt
1/4 tsp. soda
2 tsp. baking powder
1/3 c. corn oil
2/3 c. salt free peanut butter
1/4 c. Eggbeaters and 1 egg
3 tbsp. skim milk
4 tbsp. liquid sweetener
2 tbsp. sugar substitute

Sift flour, salt, soda, and baking powder. Cream next 6 ingredients together add oatmeal, beat. Add flour mixture, stir until it forms a ball; roll into 1 inch balls. Place on ungreased cookie sheet. Press down with glass. Bake at 375 degrees for 10 minutes. approx 35 calories per cookie.

DIABETIC PEANUT BUTTER COOKIES

1 c. flour
1/2 c. creamy peanut butter
1 egg
1 tsp. vanilla
1/4 tsp. salt
1 1/2 tsp. baking powder
1/2 c. water
1 tbsp. liquid sweetener
1/2 c. salad oil

Mix all together in a large bowl. Shape into balls and place on ungreased cookie sheet. Bake at 375 degrees for 12 to 15 minutes. (You may add a little more flour if desired.)

DIABETIC PEANUT BUTTER COOKIES

1/3 c. plain flour
1/4 tsp. baking soda
1/4 tsp. baking powder
Pinch of salt
2 tbsp. shortening
2 tbsp. peanut butter
1 tsp. Sweet 'n Low
1 egg, beaten

Mix and stir all ingredients in order (flour, baking soda, baking powder, salt, shortening, peanut butter and Sweet 'n Low). Add beaten egg and mix well. Drop by large teaspoon on greased cookie sheet. Bake at 350 degrees for 10 minutes.

DIABETIC FUDGE

1 14 1/2 oz. evaporated milk
3 tbsp. cocoa
1/4 c. oleo
Liquid Sweetner to equal 1/2 c. sugar
1/4 tsp. salt
1 tsp. vanilla
2 1/2 c. graham cracker crumbs
1/4 c. nuts

Combine milk and cocoa in saucepan. Beat well. Add oleo, sweetner, salt. Bring to boil. Remove from heat. Stir in remaining ingredients except 1/4 cup graham crackers. Cool about 15 minutes. Divide mixture into 32 balls. Roll in remaining cracker crumbs and chill.

PINEAPPLE SHERBET (FOR DIABETICS)

1 (16 oz.) can crushed pineapple in pineapple juice
1 tsp. unflavored gelatin (1/3 envelope)
2 tbsp. lemon juice nonnutritive sweetener equivalent to 1/2 cup sugar
1/2 c. nonfat dry milk powder

At least 3 1/2 hours before serving: Drain pineapple, reserving juice. In small saucepan, into 1/4 cup reserved pineapple juice, sprinkle gelatin. Cook over low heat, stirring constantly until gelatin is dissolved. Remove from heat; stir in 1/2 cup reserved pineapple juice, lemon juice, crushed pineapple and nonnutritive sweetener; cool.   In small bowl with mixer at high speed, beat milk powder with 1/2 cup ice water until stiff peaks form; gently stir in gelatin mixture until well combined. Pour into shallow pan; freeze 3 hours or until firm. Makes 8 servings.

ORANGE SHERBET (FOR DIABETICS)

1 c. orange juice
1 tsp. unflavored gelatin (1/3 envelope)
2 tbsp. lemon juice
1 tbsp. grated orange peel nonnutritive sweetener equal to 1/2 cup sugar
1/2 c. nonfat dry milk powder

Mix all ingredients together until well blended.

DIABETIC APPLE PIE

Pastry for 8 inch two crust pie
6 c. sliced tart apples
3/4 tsp. cinnamon or nutmeg
1 (12 oz.) can frozen Seneca apple juice
2 tbsp. cornstarch

Heat oven to 425 degrees. Put apples in pastry lined pan. Heat juice, cornstarch and spice (optional). Let it boil until clear. Pour over apples. Cover with top crust. Bake 50 to 60 minutes.

DIABETIC'S PUMPKIN PIE

1 baked, cooked 9 inch pie shell
2 sm. pkgs. sugar free instantvanilla pudding c. milk

1 c. canned pumpkin
1 tsp. pumpkin pie spice
1/4 tsp. nutmeg
1/4 tsp. ginger
1/2 tsp. cinnamon

Blend all ingredients in blender until smooth. Use plain canned pumpkin. Do not use canned pumpkin pie mixture. Pour into pie shell and chill until ready to serve.

SUGAR-FREE DIABETIC CAKE

2 c. raisins
2 c. water
2 eggs, lightly beaten (you can use eggbeaters or egg whites)
1 tsp. vanilla extract
1/2 c. skim milk
2 c. unsweetened applesauce
3 tsp. Sweet & Low
1 tsp. cinnamon
1 tsp. nutmeg
1 tsp. salt
1 tsp. baking powder
2 c. all-purpose flour
1 c. chopped nuts (optional)

You may substitute the nuts with 1/2 cup mashed bananas for a uniquely different flavor, if so, mix banana with the wet ingredients. Preheat oven to 350 degrees. Cook raisins in water until all water is absorbed, about 30 minutes. Mix all the wet ingredients in one bowl and all the dry ingredients in a separate bowl. The nuts get added to the flour mixture then add the flour mixture to the liquid mixture. Fold in the raisins. Bake in loaf or bundt pan for 35 to 45 minutes or until toothpick inserted comes out clean.

STRAWBERRY DIABETIC JAM

1 c. berries
3/4 c. sugar-free strawberry pop
1 pkg. strawberry sugar-free Jello
3 packets Equal

Mash the berries, add soda pop and cook 1 minute. Remove from heat and stir in Jello until dissolved. Stir in sweetener and pour in jars. Seal and store in refrigerator. Yields about 1 1/4 cups. You may use other fruits such as raspberries, peaches or cherries.

DIABETIC PUNCH

1-2 liter diet Sprite
1 (46 oz.) can chilled unsweetened pineapple juice
1 pkg. blueberry Kool-Aid with Nutrasweet

Chill all ingredients and pour in punch bowl and serve.

DIABETIC EGG NOG

1 1/2 c. milk
5 sucaryl tablets
4 eggs, beaten well
2 tsp. vanilla

Put all ingredients together and mix well.

DIABETIC JELLY

1 qt. sugarless apple juice
4 tbsp. artificial sweetener (can add more)
4 tbsp. lemon juice
2 pkg. unflavored gelatin

Mix ingredients and boil gently for 5 minutes. Cool and pour into containers. Store in refrigerator.

DIABETIC COOKIES

1 c. raisins
1 c. water
2 eggs, beaten
1 tsp. vanilla
1 c. flour
1/4 c. dates, chopped
1/2 c. shortening
3 tsp. sweetener
1 tsp. soda

Boil raisins, dates and water for 3 minutes. Add shortening and cool. Add eggs, then all remaining ingredients and mix well. Chill. Drop onto ungreased cookie sheet. Bake at 350 degrees for 10 to 12 minutes.

DIABETIC FRUIT COOKIES

1 c. flour
1 tsp. baking soda
1 c. water
1 c. dates, chopped
1/2 c. apples, peeled & chopped
3/4 c. raisins
1/2 c. margarine
1 c. quick oats
2 eggs, beaten (or eggbeaters)
1 tsp. vanilla
1 c. pecans, chopped

Sift flour and soda, set aside. Cook water, dates, apple and raisins; bring to a boil. Simmer 3 minutes. Remove from heat and add the margarine and stir. Cool mixture and then add eggs, oatmeal and the dry ingredients; add the vanilla and nuts. Cover and refrigerate overnight. Drop on cookie sheets 2 inches apart. Bake in 350 degree oven for about 24 minutes. Store in the refrigerator in air tight container. May also add 1 tsp. cinnamon to dry ingredients if desired.

NO BAKE DIABETIC FRUIT CAKE

1 lb. graham crackers, crushed (reserve 3 double crackers)
1/2 lb. margarine
1 lb. marshmallows

Melt above and add cracker crumbs. 3/4 c. grated raisins 1 tsp. coconut flavoring 1/2 c. dried apricots 1/2 c. raw cranberries 3/4 c. dates, cut up   Add to first mixture and mix well. Pat mixture in 6"x13"x2" pan lined with plastic wrap. Chill.

DIABETIC RAISIN CAKE

2 c. water
2 c. raisins

Cook until water evaporates. Add: 2 eggs 2 tbsp. sweetener 3/4 c. cooking oil 1 tsp. soda 2 c. flour 1 1/2 tsp. cinnamon 1 tsp. vanilla Mix well. Pour into 8"x8" greased pan, bake at 350 degrees for 2 minutes. Makes 20 servings. 1 fruit, 2 fat, 185 calories.

DIABETIC SPONGE CAKE

7 eggs
1/2 c. fruit juice, orange
3 tbsp. Sweet 'n Low or any sugar substitute
2 tbsp. lemon juice
3/4 tsp. cream of tartar
1 1/2 c. sifted cake flour
1/4 tsp. salt

Separate eggs. Beat egg whites with salt until foamy. Add cream of tartar and continue beating until stiff. In another bowl, combine rest of ingredients and mix well. Fold in beaten egg whites. Bake in greased and floured bundt pan at 350 degrees for 40 minutes or longer; test with toothpick. Serve with no sugar jelly (all fruit) and Cool Whip.

DIABETIC ORANGE DATE BARS

1 c. chopped dates
1/4 c. sugar
1/3 c. vegetable oil
1/2 c. orange juice
1 c. all purpose flour
1/2 c. chopped pecans
1 egg
1 1/2 tsp. baking powder
1 tbsp. grated orange rind

Combine dates, sugar, oil and juice in a saucepan. Cook for 5 minutes to soften dates. Cool. Add remaining ingredients. Spread into an oiled 8"x8" baking pan. Bake in 350 degree oven for 25 to 30 minutes. Cool before cutting. Makes 36 bars.

DATE DIABETIC COOKIES

2/3 c. cold water
3/4 c. oleo
1 c. chopped dates
1 egg
1/4 tsp. nutmeg
1 tbsp. cinnamon
1/2 tsp. soda
1/2 tsp. baking powder
1 tbsp. sweetener
1 tbsp. water
1 c. flour

Cook cold water, oleo and dates for 3 to 4 minutes and cool. Mix all ingredients. Drop by teaspoons on greased cookie sheet. Bake at 350 degrees for 12 minutes or until done.

SUGARLESS COOKIES (FOR DIABETICS)

1 c. flour
1 1/2 tsp. cinnamon
1 tsp. baking soda
1/2 tsp. salt (opt.)
1/4 tsp. nutmeg
1 tsp. ground cloves
1 tsp. allspice
1 1/2 c. raisins
1 c. unsweetened applesauce
1/2 c. oil
2 eggs
1 tsp. vanilla
1/2 c. chopped nuts
1 c. quick (Mother's) oats

Mix dry ingredients and add remaining ingredients to moisten. Drop by teaspoonful onto greased cookie sheet. Bake at 375 degrees for 12 minutes.

DIABETIC NUT LOAF

24 or 2 1/2 c. dates or raisins
2 eggs
1/4 c. vegetable oil
2 c. flour, self rising
1/2 c. chopped nuts
1 tsp. baking soda
2 tsp. liquid sweetener
1 tsp. vanilla

If using all purpose flour, add 1/2 teaspoon salt and 1 teaspoon baking powder. Use 350 degree oven. Put cut dates or raisins into bowl; sprinkle with baking soda and cover with 1 cup boiling water. Let stand until cool.

DIABETIC DATE CAKE

1 stick oleo or margarine
1 egg
2 c. flour
2 tsp. soda
1 tsp. vanilla
1 c. dates
2/3 c. Sugar Twin
1/2 tsp. cinnamon
1/4 tsp. cloves
1 1/2 c. applesauce
1 c. nuts

Cream oleo; add egg, sugar and vanilla and sift together. Add dry ingredients. Add dates, applesauce and nuts. Beat at medium speed until blended. Bake one hour at 350 degrees.

DIABETIC APPLESAUCE COOKIES

1 3/4 c. cake flour
1 tsp. cinnamon
1/2 tsp. nutmeg
1/2 tsp. cloves
1 tsp. baking powder
Salt (opt.)
1/2 c. butter
1 tbsp. Sweet Ten
1 egg
1 c. unsweetened applesauce
1/2 c. raisins or nuts
1 c. All Bran

Mix ingredients. Drop on cookie sheet. Bake 20 minutes at 375 degrees.

DIABETIC HEALTH COOKIES

1 c. raisins
1/2 c. chopped dates
1/2 c. chopped apples
1 c. water
1/2 c. vegetable shortening
2 well beaten eggs
2 tsp. artificial sweetener (such as sweet n low)
1 tsp. vanilla
1 tsp. baking soda
1 c. flour
3/4 c. chopped nuts

Boil raisins, dates, and apples in water for 3 minutes. Add shortening to melt, then cool and add rest of ingredients with the nuts last. Mix well. Drop by teaspoons onto cookie sheet. Bake at 350 degrees for 10 to 12 minutes. Store in refrigerator in an airtight container.

MARY TYLER MOORE'S ALMOND MERINGUE COOKIES (DIABETIC)

4 egg whites
8 tsp. powdered skim milk
1 tsp. vanilla extract
1 tsp. almond extract
1 tsp. liquid artificial sweetner
Cinnamon to taste

Beat egg whites until stiff. Add skim milk powder. Mix well. Add extracts and sugar substitute. Drop cookies by spoonfuls onto cookie sheet. Bake at 275 degrees for 45 minutes. Remove from cookie sheet and dust with cinnamon. Yields 2 to 2 1/2 dozen. One cookie equals 32 calories.

DIABETIC BARS

1/2 c. dates
1/2 c. raisins
1/2 c. prunes
3 eggs
1/2 c. oleo or margarine
1 tsp. soda
1 tsp. vanilla
1/4 tsp. salt
1 c. flour

Cut up fruits and boil with 1 cup water add margarine. Mix all the other ingredients with eggs and dry ingredients. Add fruit mixture. Bake in greased 9 inch square pan at 350 degrees for 25 to 30 minutes. *NOTE: 1/4 teaspoon each cinnamon and nutmeg may be added *Optional- 1/2 cup nuts or coconut may be used*.

DIABETIC COOKIES

1 c. seedless raisins
2 c. water
12 saccharin tablets
1 c. flour
1/2 c. shortening
1 tsp. cinnamon
1/2 tsp. nutmeg
1/2 tsp. cloves
1 tsp. soda
1 tsp. vanilla
1 c. quick oats

Cook raisins in water for 15 minutes, adding saccharin while hot. Sift dry ingredients. Mix all together, drop on cookie sheet and flatten. Bake at 350 degrees for 15 minutes. Keep refrigerated.

BANANA NUT SQUARES FOR DIABETICS

2/3 c. margarine
4 pkg. Sweet 'n Low or 2 or 3 tsp.
2 eggs, separated (stiffly beat whites)
1 c. mashed bananas
1 1/2 c. flour
1 tsp. baking soda
1/4 tsp. baking powder
1/4 tsp. salt
1/4 c. sour cream
1/2 tsp. vanilla
1/2 c. chopped nuts

Cream Sweet 'n Low and margarine. Add egg yolks and mix well. Add bananas, sift dry ingredients. Add alternately with sour cream to shortening mixture. Mix until well blended. Add vanilla, stiffly beaten egg whites and nuts. Pour into two 8x8 or 9x9 inch square pans. Doesn't rise like regular bars.

DIABETIC AND LOW SODIUM POUND CAKE

2 c. flour
1/2 c. corn oil
2 eggs
3 lg. ripe bananas
1 1/2 tbsp. liquid sweetener
4 tbsp. buttermilk
1 c. raisins
1 tsp. soda
1 tsp. vanilla
1 1/2 c. pecans

Pre-heat oven to 300 degrees Sift flour and soda together. Add oil, liquid sweetener and mix well until light. Beat in eggs. Add rest of ingredients. Beat until well mixed. Pour into loaf pan. Bake at 350 degrees for 25 minutes

----

DIABETIC BREAD PUDDING

1 slice white bread, cut in cubes
2 or 3 tbsp. raisins
1 c. skim milk
1 egg, well beaten
2 pkgs. artificial sweetener
1 tsp. vanilla

Beat egg, milk, vanilla and sweetener together. Spray two (2) cup microwave dish with non-sticking vegetable spray. Arrange bread cubes and raisins in dish. Pour milk mixture over bread to moisten each cube. Sprinkle dash of nutmeg over top and microwave on high for five (5) minutes or until knife inserted in center comes out clean. Be careful not to overcook.

DIABETIC HEALTH COOKIES

1 c. raisins
1/2 c. chopped dates
1/2 c. chopped apples
1 c. water
1/2 c. vegetable shortening
2 well beaten eggs
2 pkgs. Sweet & Low (optional)
1 tsp. vanilla
1 tsp. baking soda
1 c. flour
3/4 c. chopped nuts

Boil raisins, dates and apples in water for 3 minutes. Add shortening to melt. Cool, then add rest of ingredients. Add nuts last. Mix well. Drop by teaspoons onto cookie sheet. Bake at 350 degrees for 10 to 12 minutes. Store in refrigerator in an airtight container.

APPLESAUCE DIABETIC COOKIES

1/2 c. flour
1 tsp. cinnamon
1/2 tsp. soda
1/4 tsp. allspice
1/2 c. quick rolled oats
1/2 c. raisins
1/2 c. unsweetened applesauce
1 egg, beaten
1/4 c. shortening
2 tsp. vanilla
Optional: 1/4 tsp. orange flavoring, nuts

Mix moist ingredients first then add dry ingredients. Drop on greased baking sheet. Bake at 350 degrees for 8 to 10 minutes. Yield: 1 1/2 dozen.

BIRTHDAY CAKE FOR DIABETIC

2 c. sifted cake flour
2 1/2 tsp. baking powder
1/2 tsp. salt
6 tbsp. softened margarine
1 1/4 tsp. vanilla
1/4 tsp. almond extract
1 c. sugar
1 egg
3/4 c. milk
1/2 c. sugar-free strawberry jam
1 c. nondairy whipped topping

Preheat oven to 350 degrees. Line two 8 inch round cake pans with parchment paper or waxed paper. Sift together the flour, baking powder and salt. With an electric mixer at medium speed, cream together margarine, vanilla and almond extract until fluffy. Gradually add sugar, beating constantly. Add egg; beat until mixture is fluffy. stirring with a spoon, add the dry ingredients alternately with milk. Stirring after each addition until batter is smooth. Pour into the prepared pans. Bake 25-30 minutes or until done. When cool spread the strawberry jam between the layers. Spread whipped topping on the top. Store in refrigerator until just before serving. For added color you can add a drop of (your color choice) food coloring to the whipped topping before putting it on top of cake.

DIABETIC CAKE

1 c. raisins
1 1/2 c. water
1/2 c. shortening
1 egg
1 c. oatmeal
1 tbsp. sugar substitute
1 c. flour
1 tsp. baking soda
1/4 tsp. salt
1/2 tsp. cinnamon

Boil raisins and water. Add other ingredients. Bake in a loaf pan at 350 degrees about 45 minutes or until done.

DIABETIC COOKIES

1 1/2 c. unsweetened applesauce
3/4 c. margarine
2 eggs
1 tbsp. vanilla
1/3 c. brown sugar substitute, suitable for baking
2 c. oatmeal
1 tbsp. cinnamon
1/2 tsp. allspice
1 1/2 c. flour
1 1/2 tsp. soda
1/2 tsp. salt
1 c. raisins
1/4 c. nuts

Mix applesauce, margarine, eggs, vanilla and brown sugar substitute well; add the remaining ingredients. Drop by teaspoonfuls onto a cookie sheet and bake at 375 degrees for 15 minutes.

DIABETIC FRUIT CAKES

2 c. water
2 c. raisins
1 c. unsweetened apple sauce
2 eggs
2 tbsp. liquid sweetener
3/4 c. cooking oil
1 tsp. soda
2 c. plain flour
1 1/4 tsp. cinnamon
1/2 tsp. nutmeg
1 tsp. vanilla

Cook raisins in water until water is gone. Add the applesauce, eggs, sweetener and oil and mix well. Blend in the other ingredients which have been sifted together. Add vanilla. Pour into greased and floured pans, preferably loaf pans. Bake about 1 hour at 350 degrees or until done. Makes 10 to 12 servings.

DIABETIC PEANUT BUTTER COOKIES

1/2 c. peanut butter
1 tbsp. low calorie oleo
2 1/2 tsp. liquid sweetener
2 eggs
1 c. flour
1/4 tsp. soda
1/2 c. skimmed milk

Beat first 4 ingredients well. Add eggs and beat again, then add milk and flour. Blend well. Drop by spoon on cookie sheet that is greased well. Bake at 375 degrees for 12 minutes.

DIABETIC COOKIES

1 egg
1/2 c. margarine, melted
2 tsp. cinnamon
1 c. flour
1 c. quick-rolled oats
1 c. applesauce
1 c. raisins
1 tsp. soda
3 pkgs. sugar substitute

Place all ingredients in bowl and mix well. Drop by teaspoons on cookie sheet and bake for 10 to 12 minutes at 375 degrees. *Makes about 3 dozen.*

DIABETIC CAKE

2 c. diced apples, cooked
2 eggs
1 c. nuts
1/2 tsp. cinnamon
1 tsp. soda
1/2 c. Sugar Twin
3/4 c. butter
1 c. raisins
2 c. flour
1/2 tsp. salt

Mix all ingredients together in order above. Bake in tube pan 1 hour at 350 degrees.

DIABETIC CAKE

1 c. raisins cooked in 1 c. water
1 c. prunes, cooked in 1 c. water, cut up
1 c. unsweetened applesauce
2 eggs

1/4 c. Sweet-n-Low
3/4 c. Wesson oil
2 c. self-rising flour
1 tsp. vanilla
1 tsp. cinnamon
1 tsp. nutmeg
1 tsp. soda
1 c. black walnuts, chopped

Dredge walnuts and raisins in flour. Beat eggs and applesauce together. Combine all other ingredients and bake at 350 degrees for 35-40 minutes in sheet pan.

DIABETIC COOKIES

1 box raisins
2 c. water
1 1/2 sticks butter
3 eggs
1 tsp. vanilla
1 1/2 tsp. baking powder
1 1/2 tsp. soda dissolved in 3 tsp. water
1 tsp. cinnamon
Pinch of salt

Boil together raisins, water and butter about 2 minutes. When cool, add eggs, Sweet-N-Low, vanilla and soda. Sift together flour, salt, cinnamon, baking powder. Add to first cooked mixture. Add 1 cup nuts, if desired. Drop on greased cookie sheet and bake about 20 minutes at 350 degrees.

DIABETIC CAKE

1 c. raisins, cooked in 1 c. water, cool
1 c. prunes, cut up, cook in 1 c. water, cool
1 c. applesauce, sweet or unsweetened
2 eggs
1/4 c. Sweet-N-Low
3/4 c. corn oil
2 c. self-rising flour

1 tsp. vanilla
1 tsp. cinnamon
1 tsp. nutmeg
1 tsp. soda
1 c. chopped pecans or black walnuts
Dredge nuts and raisins in flour. Beat egg and applesauce. Combine all ingredients and bake at 350 degrees for 35-40 minutes in shallow pan.

DIABETIC BROWNIES

2 c. graham cracker crumbs (approximately 24 crackers)
1/2 c. chopped walnuts
3 oz. semi-sweet chocolate
1 1/2 tsp. Sweet-N-Low (6 packs)
1/4 tsp. salt
1 c. skim milk

Heat oven to 350 degrees. Place all ingredients in bowl; blend well. Bake in greased 8x8x2 pan for 30 minutes. Cut in 2-inch squares while warm.

DIABETIC SPICE CAKE

1/2 c. margarine
3 eggs, beaten
1 1/2 c. unsweetened applesauce
1 c. raisins
1/2 tsp. vanilla
2 tsp. soda
1 tbsp. Artificial sweetner
1 c. dates, chopped fine
3 apples, peeled and cut in lg. pieces
1 tsp. cinnamon
2 c. flour
1 c. pecans, chopped

Mix all ingredients and bake in prepared Bundt pan (spray with Pam) in 350 degree oven for 1 hour.

DIABETIC CAKE

2 c. raisins
2 c. water
1 c. unsweetened applesauce
2 eggs
3/4 c. oil
2 tbsp. liquid sweetener
2 c. flour
1/4 tsp. nutmeg
1 tsp. soda
1 tsp. vanilla

Cook raisins in water until water is gone. Add next 4 ingredients to raisins after they cool. Mix well. Sift dry ingredients together and add. Add vanilla, mix well. Pour into a greased loaf pan. Bake 1 hour or longer at 350 degrees.

DIABETIC OATMEAL COOKIES

1/2 c. margarine
1 egg
1 tsp. sucaryl solution
1/4 c. milk
1 c. flour
1/2 tsp. baking powder
1/8 tsp. baking soda
1 tsp. cinnamon
1/2 tsp. nutmeg
1/4 tsp. salt
1 tsp. vanilla
1/2 c. raisins
1 c. rolled oats

Cream margarine. Add beaten egg, sucaryl solution, and milk. Sift and mix dry ingredients and then add to first mixture. Beat in vanilla, raisins, and rolled oats. Drop by teaspoon onto greased cookie sheet and bake. You can use 1/4 cup margarine and 1/4 cup applesauce or 1 banana instead of using the full amount of margarine.

DATE NUT COOKIES (DIABETIC)

1/2 c. softened oleo or margarine
1 tsp. liquid sweetener
2 tsp. water
1/2 tsp. vanilla
1 beaten egg
1 c. plus 2 tbsp. flour
1/2 tsp. soda
1/2 tsp. salt
1/2 c. chopped dates
1/2 c. chopped nuts

Cream butter, add sweetener, water, vanilla and beaten egg. Sift dry ingredients and add to mixture. Bake on greased cookie sheet 10-12 minutes at 375 degrees.

ANN'S DIABETIC COFFEE CAKE

1 c. flour
1/2 c. margarine
2 tbsp. water

Mix and roll dough into ball, divide into 2 balls. Place onto ungreased cookie sheet. Pat down, 12 inches long - 3 inches wide.
--FILLING--

1/2 c. margarine
1 c. water
1 tsp. almond extract
1 c. flour
3 eggs

Mix margarine and water in saucepan. Bring to a boil and add flavoring, then remove from heat. Add flour, then add eggs one at a time. Divide into half. Spread on dough, one then the other. Bake at 350 degrees for 60 minutes.

DIABETIC APPLESAUCE LOAF CAKE

3 c. flour
1 1/2 c. sugar substitute
2 tsp. baking soda
2 tsp. baking powder
2 tsp. cinnamon
1/2 tsp. salt
2 c. applesauce, unsweetened
1 c. oil
4 eggs
1 c. raisins
1/2 c. chopped walnuts
1 c. chopped dates

Combine all ingredients. Pour batter into 2 ungreased 9 x 6 x 4 inch loaf pans. Bake at 350 degrees for 45 minutes.

DIABETIC CHOCOLATE CHIP COOKIES

1/4 c. margarine, softened
1 1/2 tsp. vanilla
1 c. + 2 tbsp. flour
2 tsp. baking powder
1/2 c. semi-sweet chocolate chips
1/4 c. chopped nuts
4 tsp. liquid sweetener
1 egg
1/2 tsp. salt
1/4 tsp. soda

Combine first 4 ingredients in small mixer bowl. Beat at high speed for 1 to 2 minutes or until light and fluffy. Add next 4 ingredients with 1/2 cup water. Blend at low speed until well combined. Stir in chocolate chips and nuts. Dough will be soft. Drop onto ungreased cookie sheet. Bake at 425 degrees for 10 to 12 minutes.

DIABETIC JELLY

1 c. unsweetened juice (any kind)
1/4 tsp. lemon juice
2 tbsp. sugar substitute
1 tbsp. plain gelatin
1 tbsp. cornstarch

Mix lemon juice, sugar substitute, gelatin and cornstarch. Add fruit juice and stir well to mix. Boil hard for 3 minutes, stirring constantly. Makes 1 small jar. Store in refrigerator.

DIABETIC APPLE JELLY

2 env. unflavored gelatin
2 c. unsweetened apple juice
Artificial sweetener to taste
2 tbsp. lemon juice
Yellow food coloring

Sterilize 2 half-pint jars by covering with water and boiling for 15 minutes. Soften gelatin in 1 cup apple juice. Heat to a boil the other cup of apple juice. Remove from heat. Add juice with softened gelatin. Add lemon juice. Bring to full boil and cook about 2 minutes. Remove from heat and add food coloring and sweetener to taste. Pour into sterile half-pint jars, seal, and cool. Store in refrigerator. Makes 2 half-pints.

DIABETIC SPAGHETTI SAUCE

1 tsp. vegetable oil 1 1/4 lb. lean ground round 3 (8 oz.) cans tomato sauce 1 (6 oz.) can tomato paste 4 c. water 1/4 tsp. salt (optional) 1 tsp. pepper 1 tsp. oregano Dash of garlic Brown onions in oil; add meat and brown. Drain fat; add rest of ingredients. Simmer 1 hour uncovered. Serving size, 1/2 cup. (Lean meat exchange 1, vegetable exchange 1, Calories 90, Carbohydrates 5 g, Protein 7 g, Fat 5 g, Fiber 0 g, Cholesterol 21 mg, Sodium 264 mg.

DIABETIC BARBECUE SAUCE

1 sm. onion, minced
1 (8 oz.) can tomato sauce
2 c. water
1/4 c. wine vinegar
1/4 c. Worcestershire sauce
1 tsp. salt (optional)
2 tsp. paprika
2 tsp. chili powder
1 tsp. pepper
1/2 tsp. cinnamon
1/8 tsp. cloves

Combine all ingredients; bring to full boil. Simmer 20 minutes.
Serving size = 1/4 cup

ANNE'S DIABETIC CHOCOLATE SYRUP

1/3 c. dry cocoa
1 1/4 c. cold water
1/4 tsp. salt
2 tsp. vanilla
3 tsp. liquid sweetner

Combine all ingredients; bring to full boil. Simmer 20 minutes.

DIABETIC CINNAMON COOKIES

1 slice bread, crumbled
1/4 tsp. cinnamon
1/4 tsp. vanilla
1 egg, beaten
1 tsp. sweetener

Mix all ingredients together, drop on cookie sheet, bake at 350
degrees for about 10 - 15 min or until lightly brown.

DIABETIC NUT COOKIES

1/2 c. flour
1/4 tsp. baking powder
1/8 tsp. salt
1/2 tsp. Sweet and Low
2 tbsp. unsweetened orange juice
1/2 tsp. vanilla
2 tbsp. vegetable shortening
2 tbsp. chopped nuts
2 tbsp. grated orange rind

Mix all ingredients together, drop on cookie sheet, bake at 350 degrees for about 10 - 15 min or until lightly brown.

DIABETIC EASTER FUDGE

1 sq. unsweetened chocolate
1/4 c. evaporated milk
1/2 tsp. vanilla
1 tsp. artificial liquid sweetener
1 pkg. vanilla or chocolate sweetened pudding powder
8 tsp. finely chopped nuts

Mix all ingredients together and bring to a boil over med. heat, stirring constantly. When mixture begins to thicken , quickly pour into pan or dish to cool and set. May be refrigerated to hasten cooling.

SPICED TEA (DIABETIC)

1 c. instant tea with NutraSweet
2 pkg. Kool aid
Sunshine Punch with NutraSweet
1 tsp. cinnamon
1 tsp. cloves

 Add desired portion to cup of hot water.

DIABETIC CRANBERRY AND ORANGE SALAD

1 lb. fresh cranberries
1 med. orange, do not peel
1 med. apple, do not peel
1 lg. celery stalk

Grind the above ingredients together. 1 (3 oz.) box orange sugar free Jello 2 tbsp. Equal sweetener Dissolve Jello in 3/4 cup boiling water; add 3/4 cup cold water. Add ground fruit, celery, pineapple, sweetener. Chill.

DIABETIC GLORIFIED RICE

1/2 c. rice, uncooked (not instant)
1 (20 oz.) crushed pineapple, in own juice
1 (3 oz.) pkg. sugar-free fruit flavored gelatin
Boiling water
Pineapple juice, drained from can
Maraschino cherries
Heavy cream

Cook rice according to package directions. Drain, set aside. Drain pineapple, reserving 1 cup juice. Dissolve gelatin in 1 cup boiling water. Add juice. Stir in well drained rice, the cooked rice will absorb the color and flavor of the gelatin. Mix well and chill until thickened but not quite set. Add drained pineapple and cherries, if desired. Fold in cream that has been whipped. Chill. Makes about 8 servings.

NO CALORIE DIABETIC DRESSING

1/2 c. water
1/2 c. white vinegar
1/2 tsp. salt
1/2 tsp. dry mustard
1/8 tsp. pepper
1/16 tsp. paprika
Artificial sweetener to substitute for 4 tsp. sugar

Combine all ingredients and refrigerate. Makes about 1 cup. 1 serving = 1-2 tablespoons. *Diabetics - this is a free exchange. Sodium value 133 mg/2 tablespoons (low sodium diets omit salt). No cholesterol, protein fat or calories.

CARROT CABBAGE SLAW (DIABETIC RECIPE)

1/2 head cabbage
1 sm. onion
2 celery stalks
2 carrots
1 tbsp. mayonnaise
2 pkg. Artificial sweetner (such as sweet n low)
1/2 tsp. black pepper
2 tbsp. vinegar
2 tbsp. lemon juice

Shred cabbage and carrots. Finely chop onion and celery. Mix together in a large bowl. In a separate bowl, mix together sweetner, pepper, vinegar, lemon juice, and mayonnaise. Pour over shredded vegetables and refrigerate. Makes 10 servings. Exchanges: One serving equals 1 vegetable; calories: one serving equals 23 calories.

DIABETIC CREAM CHEESE SALAD

1 (3 oz.) env. sugar free Jello (lime)
1 c. crushed pineapple in own juice
3 oz. lite cream cheese, room temperature
1/2 c. evaporated skim milk, chilled

Mix Jello per package directions. Drain juice from pineapple and add water to make 1/2 cup liquid. Add juice to Jello mixture and chill until syrupy.   Beat the evaporated skim milk, making sure that the bowl, beaters and milk are well chilled. Set whipped milk aside. Beat the cream cheese into Jello. Fold in the whipped milk and drained pineapple and chill in mold or glass dish. Makes 9 ½-cup servings.

EASY SUGAR-FREE DESSERT

1 (6 oz.) pkg. sugar-free Jello
2 c. hot water
1/2 pkg. Crystal Light lemonade mix
2 c. water
3 c. Cool Whip
1 angle food cake

Dissolve Jello in hot water. Add lemonade mix and water. Chill until slightly thickened, beat until frothy and fold in Cool Whip. Fold in cake broken in pieces. Put into 9 x 13 inch pan and chill.

CREAM PUFFS

½ Margarine
1 c. boliling water
1 c. flour
½ tsp salt
4 eggs

Melt margarine in 1 cup boiling water. Sift flour and salt together. Add to boiling liquid all at once and stir until mixture leaves side of pan in compact ball. Cool 1 minute.

Put in mixing bowl and add eggs - one at a time, beating well after each addition. Drop by rounded teaspoon onto ungreased cookie sheet. Bake at 450 degrees for 10 minutes and then at 400 degrees for about 25 minutes. Cool and fill with favorite filling. *Suggested filling: 1 tub Cool Whip, stir in 1/2 package instant vanilla pudding.*

SUGARLESS APPLE PIE

1 (12 oz.) can frozen apple juice concentrate, thawed
3 tbsp. cornstarch
1/4 tsp. salt
1 tsp. cinnamon
1/2 tsp. nutmeg
5-6 apples, peeled, cored and sliced

Mix all ingredients, bring to a boil. Pour into crust-lined pie plate. Top with remaining crust. Bake at 425 degrees about 45 minutes until crust is golden and apples are tender.

SUGAR-FREE SPICE COOKIES

1/3 c. margarine, softened
1/4 c. granulated fructose
1/2 tsp. granulated brown sugar replacement
1 c. flour
1/2 tsp. baking powder
1 tsp. cinnamon
1/8 tsp. salt
1 tsp. vanilla

In a large bowl, cream margarine, fructose, and brown sugar replacement together until light and fluffy. Add flour, baking powder, cinnamon, and salt; mix well. Stir in vanilla. Shape dough into 1-inch balls and place on ungreased cookie sheets. Flatten balls with a fork that has been dipped in cold water. Bake at 375 degrees for 8-10 minutes; cool on wire racks.

GRILLED TURKEY TENDERLOIN

1/4 c. low-sodium soy sauce
1/4 c. sherry wine or apple juice
1/8 tsp. black pepper
2 tbsp. crushed onion
1 lb. uncooked turkey tenderloin, 3/4 to 1 inch thick
1/4 c. peanut oil
2 tbsp. lemon juice
1/8 tsp. garlic salt
1/4 tsp. ground ginger

In a shallow pan, blend all marinade ingredients together. Add turkey, turning to coat both sides. Cover; marinate in refrigerator several hours or overnight, turning occasionally. Grill the tenderloins over hot coals, 8-10 minutes per side, depending on the thickness. Tenderloins

are done when there is no pink in the center - do not over cook.
Serve in 1/4 inch thick slices in toasted buns. Yields 4 servings.

DIABETIC COOKIES

1/2 c. oleo
2 tsp. sweetener
1 tsp. salt
1 egg
2 tsp. grated orange peel
1/2 c. milk
1/2 tsp. baking powder
1/2 tsp. soda
1 c. nut meats
1 1/4 c. flour

Cream oleo, sweetener, and part of flour. Stir in rest of ingredients.
Bake at 350 degrees for 10-12 minutes.

DIABETIC FRUIT BARS

1 c. chopped dates
1/2 chopped dried apricots
1/2 c. walnuts
1 1/2 tsp. baking powder
1/2 c. butter
1 1/3 c. rolled oats
1/4 c. oil
2 eggs
1 tsp. vanilla
1 c. flour
1 tsp. cinnamon

In saucepan, melt oil and butter, add dates and apricots. Remove
from heat and beat in egg and vanilla. Combine dry ingredients and
mix with rest of mixture. Bake in 9 x 13 inch pan for 20 minutes at
350 degrees.

SMAKEROON COOKIES

3 egg whites
1/2 tsp. cream of tartar
2 tsp. sugar substitute
1/4 tsp. almond flavoring
3 c. Rice Krispies
1/4 c. shredded coconut

Beat egg whites until foamy, add cream of tartar and continue beating until stiff but not dry. Add sugar substitute and flavoring. Beat until blended. Fold in cereal and coconut and drop by teaspoonfuls onto lightly greased cookie sheet. Bake at 350 degrees for 12-15 minutes or until lightly browned. 1 serving = 1 fruit exchange (3 cookies). Yields 24 cookies.

CHOCOLATE CAKE

1/4 c. sifted all purpose flour
1 tsp. baking powder
1/4 tsp. salt
3 tbsp. cocoa
1/4 c. cold coffee
1 tbsp. sugar substitute
1 egg
1 tbsp. salad oil
1/4 c. cold water
1 tsp. vanilla

Sift flour, baking powder, soda, and salt together. Blend cocoa and coffee. Beat egg and all sugar substitute, water, salad oil, and vanilla and stir into dry ingredients, mixing only until smooth. Stir in cocoa and coffee mixture. Line one 8 inch round layer cake pan with wax paper and grease with 1/8 teaspoon butter. Pour batter into pan, cover pan with foil and place in shallow pan of water. Bake at 350 degrees for 25 minutes. Remove from pan onto cake rack and cool. Cut layer in half crosswise to make half of a two layer cake. One serving = 1 fruit and 1 fat exchange.

SPONGE CAKE

7 eggs
1/2 c. cold water
3 tbsp. sugar substitute
1/2 tsp. vanilla
2 tbsp. lemon juice
1/4 tsp. cream of tartar
1 1/2 c. cake flour
1/4 tsp. salt

Beat egg yolks until thick and lemon colored. Combine water, sugar substitute, vanilla, and lemon juice. Add to egg yolks beat until thick and foamy; add cream of tartar to beaten egg whites and continue beating until stiff peaks form. Fold carefully into yolk mixture. Combine sifted flour and salt. Sift a little at a time over the mixture, folding in gently. Pour into an ungreased 9 or 10 inch tube pan. Bake at 325 degrees for 1 hour and 15 minutes. One serving = 1 bread exchange.

CHOCOLATE SAUCE

1 tbsp. butter
2 tbsp. cocoa
1 tbsp. cornstarch
1 c. skim milk
2 tsp. sugar substitute
1/8 tsp. salt

Melt butter. Combine cocoa, cornstarch and salt; blend with melted butter until smooth. Add milk and sugar substitute and cook over moderate heat, stirring constantly until slightly thickened, remove from heat. Stir in vanilla. Set pan in ice water and stir until completely cold. (Sauce thickens as it cools.) One serving - (1 tablespoon) free exchange.

BUTTERSCOTCH COOKIES

1/2 tsp. baking powder
1 c. flour

Pinch of salt
1/4 c. shortening
2 tbsp. brown sugar
1 env. or 1 1/16 oz. artificiallysweetened butterscotch pudding and pie filling mix
1/4 tsp. vanilla
1 egg

Sift together salt, flour, and baking powder. Combine shortening and sugar and cream together; slowly add pudding mix, mixing thoroughly. Then add egg, beat until mixture is light and fluffy. Stir in vanilla; and then add ingredients; mixing well. Place dough on wax paper; shape into a roll about 2 inches in diameter.

Wrap in wax paper. Place in freezer for about 30 minutes or refrigerate overnight. Cut into 1/8 inch slices then place on ungreased cookie sheet. Bake at 375 degrees for 8-10 minutes. *2 cookies = 2 fruit and 1 fat exchange. Makes 24 cookies.*

MARASCHINO CHERRY - GUMDROP COOKIES

1/2 c. margarine
1/4 c. brown sugar
1 egg yolk
1 c. flour
1 1/2 tsp. vanilla extract
1/4 tsp. salt
24 sm. gum drops or 12 maraschino cherries, halved

Cream together margarine adding sugar slowly. Mix in egg yolk and vanilla extract. After sifting dry ingredients together slowly add creamed mixture. Roll into small balls and place on ungreased cookie sheet. Bake at 350 degrees for 5 minutes. After removing from oven, gently press maraschino cherry half or 1 gumdrop in the center of each cookie. Return to oven and continue baking for an additional 8-10 minutes. *2 cookies = 1 fruit exchange and 2 fat exchanges. Yields 2 dozen cookies.*

DIET 7 - UP SALAD

1 (4 serving) pkg. sugar free lemon gelatin
1 c. boiling water
6 oz. cold diet 7-Up
1 (8 oz.) (or 1/2 of 20 oz.) can drained crushed pineapple canned in its own juice (unsweetened)
1 banana, split and sliced

Dissolve gelatin in hot water. Set aside to cool slightly, then slowly add the chilled pop, pineapple, and banana pieces. Pour into an 8 inch square pan and chill until set. Add topping.
--TOPPING--

Cook over double boiler until thickened: 1 tbsp. flour Artificial Sweetener = 1/4 c. sugar 1/2 c. reserved juice 1 tbsp. low-fat margarine   Let cool, then fold in 1 envelope of prepared D-Zerta whipped topping. Spread on top of the above "set" salad. 1 serving = 2 1/2 inch square; 1 fruit and 1 fat exchanges. *Note: If this salad is doubled and a 9 x 13 inch pan is used, do not double the topping mixture. It's sufficient to cover all.*

SAUCY CRANAPPLE SALAD

1 env. unflavored gelatin
1/4 c. cold water to soften above
1 (4 serving) pkg. sugar-free raspberry gelatin
1 c. boiling water
2 c. (1/2 lb.) frozen cranberries
1 c. juice-pack unsweetened crushed pineapple* with juice
1 c. unsweetened applesauce*
5 packets artificial sweetener

Place the clean, still frozen berries in the boiling water. Return to boiling and allow berries to pop open (8 to 15 minutes). Do not stir! Soften the unflavored gelatin in the 1/4 cup cold water, then add both gelatins to the hot cranberries; stir until dissolved. Add the pineapple with juice, the applesauce, and sweetener. Do not prepare this in a gelatin mold! Stir. Pour into a 10 cup mold and chill until set. 1 serving = 1 fruit exchange (approximately 60 calories).

PINEAPPLE COLE SLAW

12 c. shredded cabbage (about 3 lbs.)
1 c. miniature marshmallows
2 lg. (20 oz.) cans prechilled* juice pack pineapple tidbits, drained

Toss with:DRESSING:

1/4 c. reserved pineapple juice
Artificial sweetener = 1/4 c. sugar
1 1/2 c. lite Miracle Whip

Mix in a blender. Mix with slaw. Just before serving, add 2 split and sliced bananas. The slices may be placed in enough pineapple juice to cover; this will prevent them from turning brown until ready to use. 1 serving = 3/4 cup: 1 veg, 3/4 fat, 1 fruit exch. About 105 cal.

DIETETIC PASTA SALAD

Corkscrew pasta
4 fresh mushrooms, sliced
1 cucumber, sliced
Kraft reduced calorie zesty Italian dressing
1 onion, sliced
1 tomato, diced
1 green pepper, chopped

Cook and rinse pasta in cold water. Mix with remaining ingredients and marinate in dressing. Chill and serve.

LASAGNA

1 c. chopped onions
1 c. sliced mushrooms
1/2 c. diced green peppers
1 tbsp. parsley flakes
1/2 tsp. each basil, oregano, chili powder
5 oz. Mozzarella cheese
1 garlic clove, minced
1 c. chopped carrots

3 c. tomatoes
1/4 tsp. dried rosemary
3 oz. grated Romano cheese
1 1/3 c. cottage cheese

Saute onions, garlic, mushrooms, carrots, and peppers until soft. Add tomatoes, parsley, basil, oregano, chili powder, rosemary, and pepper. Simmer 15 minutes. Mix together the 3 cheeses. Starting with sauce, layer with 8 cooked lasagna noodles and cheese in an 8 x 12 inch casserole. Bake at 375 degrees for 30 minutes. Makes 4 servings.

COCONUT CUSTARD PIE

4 eggs
4 tbsp. diet oleo
1 tsp. coconut extract
5 tbsp. flour
8 oz. shredded Jicama sweetener = 1/2 c. sugar
1 3/4 c. water
1 1/2 tsp. vanilla
2/3 c. dry milk
2 slices dry bread
Dash of salt

Combine all ingredients in blender, except Jicama. Fold in Jicama and pour into crust lined 10 inch pie pan. Bake at 350 degrees for 40 to 45 minutes.

SUGAR FREE APPLE PIE

4 c. sliced, pared apples (preferably yellow delicious)
1/2 c. unsweetened apple juice concentrate (do not dilute)
1 1/2 tsp. cornstarch or tapioca
1 1/2 tsp. cinnamon or apple pie spice

Mix thickener, concentrate, and spices. Pour over apple slices to coat well. Pour into crust-lined pie plate. Top with remaining crust. Bake at 425 degrees about 45 minutes until crust is golden and apples are tender. 8 servings each 220 calories. Exchanges = 1 1/2 fruit, 1 bread, 1/2 fat each serving.

DIABETIC CHEESE CAKE

2/3 c. cottage cheese
1/3 c. cold water
1/2 tsp. vanilla
1/2 c. blueberries
1/3 c. hot water
1/3 c. powdered milk and 3 pkgs. Equal
1 tsp. lemon juice
1 env. unflavored gelatin

Soften gelatin in cold water, then add hot water. Blend until smooth. Add rest of ingredients and blend again until smooth. Stir in blueberries. Chill until firm.

RHUBARB OR CRANBERRY JELLO

2 c. rhubarb
1 pkg. Jello without sugar (raspberry, cherry, or strawberry)
1 1/4 c. water

Put rhubarb in saucepan with 1 cup water. Boil until fruit is soft. Add 1 package of Jello and stir until dissolved. Add 1/4 cup cold water. Stir and pour into individual dishes or a 1 1/2 quart casserole. Chill until set. Cranberries can be used in place of rhubarb.

POPSICLES

1 (4 serving size) env. sugar-free gelatin
1 (2 qt.) env. sugar-free artificially sweetened powdered drink mix (Kool-Aid)

In a 2 quart mixing pitcher, dissolve gelatin in 1 cup hot water. Add drink powder; stir, then add 7 cups cold water. Stir. Pour into popsicle cups with handles; freeze. Flavor Suggestions: Raspberry Lemonade Orange Orange Grape Gelatin: Triple berry Lime Hawaiian pineapple Strawberry Raspberry *These pops will not melt easily because of the absence of sugar. 1 (2 ounce) popsicle = 2 to 3 calories. 5 to 6 may be eaten per day and is considered a "free" food.*

PHUDGESICLES

1 (4 serving size) box sugar-free instant pudding (favorite flavor)
3 c. reconstituted non-fat dry milk

Whip all together according to directions on pudding package. Pour into popsicle cups with handles; freeze. 1 (2 ounce) pop = approximately 20 calories. 1 per day = "free"*. *"Free" 20 calories or fewer and is not necessary to figure into a diabetic meal plan if limited to one "free" per day.

DIABETIC APPLESAUCE COOKIES

1 3/4 c. cake flour
1/2 tsp. salt
1 tsp. cinnamon
1/2 tsp. nutmeg
1/2 tsp. cloves
1 tsp. soda
1/2 c. butter
1 tbsp. sucaryl
1 egg
1 c. applesauce (unsweetened)
1/2 c. All Bran cereal
1/2 c. raisins

Mix together the flour, salt, cinnamon, nutmeg, cloves, and soda. Mix together butter, sucaryl, and egg until light and fluffy. Add flour mixture and applesauce alternately, mixing well after each addition. Fold in raisins and All Bran. Drop on greased cookie sheet. Heat oven to 375 degrees. Bake for 20 minutes or until golden brown.

DIABETIC SPICE OATMEAL COOKIES

1 c. water
2 c. raisins
4 tbsp sweetner
½ c butter
½ tsp salt
¼ tsp allspice
½ tsp cinnamon
1 tsp soda
1/8 tsp nutmeg
2 ½ c oatmeal
½ c chopped nuts

Boil water and raisins. Cool for 5 minutes. Add all the other ingredients. Form into balls and bake on lightly greased cookie sheet for 15 minutes at 325 degrees.

DIABETIC COOKIES

1 3/4 c. flour
1 tsp. cinnamon
1/2 tsp. nutmeg
1/2 tsp. cloves
1 tsp. baking soda
1/2 c. margarine
1/2 c. Sugar Twin
1 egg
1 c. unsweetened applesauce
1/2 c. raisins, chopped
1 c. All Bran Buds
1/2 c. finely chopped nuts

Preheat oven to 350 degrees. Sift together flour, cinnamon, nutmeg, cloves and baking soda. In large bowl, mix together margarine, artificial sweetener and egg. Mix in dry ingredients, alternating with applesauce. Fold in bran, raisins and nuts and mix thoroughly. Drop onto greased cookie sheet by tablespoons. Lightly flatten with fork, dipped in milk. Bake for 7-8 minutes.

DIABETIC PUMPKIN PIE

1 sm. pkg. sugar-free vanilla pudding
1 1/2 c. milk (whole or nonfat)
1 c. canned pumpkin
1/4 tsp. cinnamon
1/4 tsp. nutmeg
Artificial sweetener to equal 1 tsp. sugar
1 baked 8-inch pie crust

Place pudding mix in a saucepan. Gradually add milk. Cook and stir over medium heat until mixture comes to a boil. Remove from heat and add pumpkin, spices and sweetener; mix well. Pour into baked crust. Chill until firm, about 3 hours.

DIABETIC WHIPPED CREAM

1/3 c. instant nonfat dry milk
1/3 c. ice water
1/2 tsp. liquid sweetener

Chill small glass bowl and beaters. Combine ingredients and whip on high speed with mixer until consistency of whipped cream. Makes about 10 servings of 2 tablespoons.

DIABETIC PUMPKIN PIE

1 (16 oz.) can pumpkin
1 (13 oz.) can evaporated milk
2 eggs
1/4 c. Brown Sugar Twin
1/4 c. Sugar Twin
1 tsp. cinnamon
1/2 tsp. salt
1/2 tsp. nutmeg
1/4 tsp. ginger
Sesame Seed Crust

Combine all ingredients and mix well in blender. Pour into Sesame Seed Crust. Bake at 425 degrees for 15 minutes, then reduce heat to 350 degrees, and bake 35 minutes longer. Exchange per serving: 1 bread, 1/2 milk, 1 fat.

--SESAME SEED CRUST--
1 c. all-purpose flour
1/4 c. sesame seed
1/2 tsp. salt
1/2 c. plus 2 tbsp. corn oil margarine
2 or 3 tbsp. cold orange juice

Combine to make 1 (9-inch) pie shell.

DIABETIC CAKE

2 c. water
2 c. raisins
1 c. unsweetened applesauce
2 eggs
2 tbsp. liquid artificial sweetener
3/4 c. cooking oil
1 tsp. baking soda
2 c. flour
1 1/2 tsp. cinnamon
1/2 tsp. nutmeg
1 tsp. vanilla

Preheat oven to 350 degrees. Cook raisins in water until water evaporates. Add applesauce, eggs, sweetener, cooking oil and mix well. Blend in baking soda and flour. Add cinnamon, nutmeg and vanilla and mix. Pour into greased 8x8 inch cake pan and bake approximately 25 minutes or until done.

STRAWBERRY PIE (NO SUGAR)

1 baked pie shell
1 qt. strawberries
3 tbsp. cornstarch
1 (8 oz.) pkg. cream cheese

1 c. apple juice, unsweetened

Slice berries, simmer 1 cup in 2/3 cups apple juice 3 minutes. Mix cornstarch with 1/3 cup apple juice, stir in berries. Stir constantly 1 minute until thick. Spread softened cheese over pie crust, put berries on cheese, pour cooked berries on top. Garnish with whipped cream and a few berries. Chill 3 to 4 hours.

SUGAR-FREE APPLE PIE

4 c. sliced peeled apples
1/2 c. undiluted frozen apple juice concentrate
1 1/2 to 2 tsp. tapioca, cornstarch or flour
1/2 tsp. lemon juice (optional)
1/2 to 1 tsp. cinnamon, nutmeg or apple pie spice

Divide pastry into 2 parts and roll thin to fit an 8 or 9-inch plate. Set aside. Mix apples, apple juice concentrate, thickener and spice and stir until apples are well coated. Add lemon juice, if desired, to keep apples lighter-colored. Taste 1 piece of apple to check the spice. Pour into the pastry-lined pie pan and top with the second crust or pastry strips. Seal the edges and cut slits in the top crust to allow steam to escape. Bake at 425 degrees for 40-45 minutes until golden brown. Serve warm or cold. NOTE: Apples have some natural pectin, but a small amount of thickener is necessary to hold the sweet concentrate of the apples for an even flavor. *One serving (including the crust)-- 220 calories; 1 1/2 fruit exchanges; 1 bread exchange; 1 fat exchange.*

APPLE PIE (NO SUGAR)

4 c. apple
1/2 c. frozen apple juice concentrate, undiluted
2 tsp. tapioca or cornstarch
1/2 to 1 tsp. cinnamon

Mix apples and all ingredients until well coated; pour into pastry shell and top with pastry. Bake at 425 degrees for 40 to 45 minutes.

POLISH SAUSAGE STEW

1 can cream of celery soup
1/4 c. brown sugar
27 oz. can sauerkraut, drained
1 1/2 lb. polish sausage, cut in 2 inch pieces
4 med. potatoes, pared and cubed
1 c. chopped onion
4 oz. shredded Monterey Jack cheese

Cook sausage,potatoes, and onion until done. Mix soup, sugar &
sauerkraut, cook until blended. Mix with other ingredients and top with
cheese.

KRAUTRUNZA

1 link (approximately 1/4 lb.) German sausage
1 lb. ground beef
1 sm. head cabbage
1 med. onion
Salt and pepper
Yeast dough

Brown meats and add other ingredients, cook until tender. serve

----
GERMAN SAUERKRAUT

1 can Bavarian sauerkraut, partially drained
1 apple, cored and sliced
1 onion, chopped
2 or 3 slices bacon

Mix together and cook until all is tender.

POLISH BIGOS AND KLUSKI

2 lb. ground beef
3 tbsp. Crisco
2 c. diced green pepper
2 c. sliced onions
10 1/2 oz. can tomato soup
#2 can tomatoes
3/4 c. water
1 - 2 tbsp. salt
1/4 tsp. black pepper
1/8 tsp. red pepper (optional)
1/2 pkg. kluski noodles

Brown ground beef. Then add peppers, onions, cook until lightly sautéed. Cook noodles per package direction. Add the rest of the ingredients and cook until well blended. Mix sauce with noodles or let them put on their own sauce.

PATCHLINGS

5 c. flour
1 egg
1 tbsp. shortening
1 c. milk

Mix all ingredients together, drop on cookie sheet, and bake at 350 degrees for about 10 min.

WALNUT DREAMS

¼ lb margarine
1 ½ c. + 1 tbsp brown sugar
1 ½ c. chopped walnuts
2 eggs (beaten)
1 ½ tsp baking powder
1 tsp vanilla
½ c. coconut

Mix all ingredients together and blend thoroughly. Drop on cookie sheet , bake at 325 degrees until lightly brown.

SUGAR-FREE CHERRY OATS MUFFIN

1 1/4 cups unbleached flour
1 1/4 teaspoons baking powder
3/4 teaspoon baking soda
1/4 teaspoon lite (or regular) salt
2/3 cup all fruit black cherry jam
1/3 cup apple juice concentrate
1/2 cup cherry juice concentrate
2 1/2 to 3 Tablespoons canola or safflower oil
1/4 cup water
2 egg whites or 1/3 cup egg white product
1 1/2 cups thin-rolled (quick) oats

Preheat your oven to 350 degrees.Sift dry ingredients together and set aside. In a different bowl, lightly beat egg whites or eggbeaterss, and mix in all wet ingredients. Mix liquid and dry ingredients,with a fork, just enough to moisten. Next, gently fold in oats and mix well.

Fill muffin tins 3/4 full, and bake at 350 degrees for 18 to 25 minutes. Check for doneness with a toothpick, if it comes out clean, they're done. Cool about 10-15 minutes. Serve warm or at room temperature. Makes 12 muffins

----

MOM'S WIENER SOUP

4 wieners
1 onion
1 qt. milk
1 1/2 tsp. salt
4 tbsp. butter
2 tbsp. flour
2 c. cooked, diced potatoes
1/4 tsp. pepper

Brown potatoes, wieners and onions in 2tbsp butter. Mix milk, salt, pepper, flour and other 2 tbsp butter together, stir constantly until mixture boils and becomes smooth. Then mix everything together in a soup pan or pot, cook until everything is hot, then serve.

GRANDMA LOE'S SKILLET CAKE

1 3/4 c. cake flour
1 tsp. baking powder
1/4 tsp. soda
1/4 tsp. salt
1 c. sugar
1/4 c. melted margarine
1 egg
1 tsp. vanilla
Buttermilk

Put margarine in cup, add egg and fill cup with buttermilk. (Blend with dry ingredients.) (beat) Before last line - sift flour, baking powder, soda, salt and sugar into bowl. Then beat with first mixture. Pour into skillet and top with topping.
--TUITTI-FRUITTI TOPPING--
1 c. drained fruit cocktail
1/2 c. brown sugar
1/4 c. chopped walnuts
1/4 c. margarine

Spoon fruit cocktail over top of batter, sprinkle brown sugar and walnuts on top of fruit cocktail, then drizzle with melted margarine

--ALMOND PRUNE TOPPING--
1 c. cooked prunes, halved
1/2 c. brown sugar
1/4 c. slivered almonds
1/4 c. margarine

MOM'S BEEF STEW

1/4 c. ginger ale
1 tbsp. red wine vinegar
1 can consomme soup
Salt and pepper
1/4 c. flour
1 lb. lean stew meat
1/4 lb. mushrooms, sliced
2 med. potatoes, cut up
2 carrots, sliced
1 onion, sliced

Brown stew meat and sautee with onions and mushrooms. Add all ingredients into pot and cook until meat is and vegetables are tender.

IOCOA EGG PANCAKES

8 eggs, whip hard
1 tsp. salt
2 1/2 c. milk or water
1 c. flour

Mix all ingredients and pour onto grill. Cook on each side until lightly brown.

DIABETIC BEEF PASTIES

--Crust—
3/4 tsp. Salt
1/4 c. plus
2 tsp. vegetable shortening
1 egg
Water

Put flour and salt in mixing bowl. Cut in shortening. Beat egg in a measuring cup. Add water to make 1/2 cup, add to flour and mix until

well moistened. Divide dough into 6 balls. On lightly floured board, roll balls into circles between waxed paper. Then set aside.
--FILLING--
3/4 lb. coarsely ground beef (raw)
2 c. diced raw potato
3/4 c. diced raw carrot
3/4 c. diced celery
1 tsp. salt
1/4 tsp. black pepper
2 tbsp. water

Once all filling ingredients have been well mixed. Spoon on to dough, and wrap around beef. Bake at 350 degrees for about 10 – 15 min or until dough has become golden brown.

TUNA SUPREME

1 sm. can tuna, water-packed
3 hard boiled eggs, diced
1 c. American cheese, diced
2 tbsp. each chopped sweet pickles, mince onion, chopped celery and cut-up stuffed olives
1/2 c. mayonnaise or Miracle Whip

Mix all ingredients and serve on bread or lettuce leaf

DIABETIC SPICY MEATBALLS

1 lb. lean ground beef
1/2 c. chili sauce
2 tsp. prepared horseradish
1/2 c. minced onion
2 tsp. Worcestershire sauce
1/2 tsp. salt
2 tbsp. corn oil

Mix all ingredients well, roll into balls, and brown in corn oil. Drain on paper towels.

DIABETIC SPICY SAUSAGE

2 lb. extra lean ground pork
2 tsp. crushed dried sage
1 tsp. freshly ground black pepper
1 tsp. fructose
1 tsp. garlic powder
1/2 tsp. onion powder
1/2 tsp. ground mace
1/4 tsp. ground allspice
1/4 tsp. salt
1/8 tsp. ground cloves

Mix all ingredients thourghly. Then make into patties and brown until done.

PORK CHOPS & STUFFING

5 pork chops
1 box croutons, prepared to box directions, as stuffing
1/4 c. water

Brown pork chops, make sure cooked well. Serve with stuffing.

DIABETIC APPLESAUCE CAKE

2 c. raisins
2 c. water
3/4 c. oil
4 tbsp. Featherweight sweetener
2 eggs
2 c. flour
1 tsp. soda

1 1/2 tsp. cinnamon
1/2 tsp. nutmeg
1/2 tsp. salt
1/2 c. nuts (if desired)
1 c. unsweetened applesauce

Sift all dry ingredients together and set aside. In a separate bowl mix all wet ingredients. Mix wet and dry ingredients together and mix well, then fold in applesauce, nuts and raisins. Pour in a greased and floured cake pan unless using a non-stick pan. Bake at 350 degrees for 25 –30 minutes or until cake springs back when lightly touched in the middle.

BANANA BREAD

2 c. all purpose flour
1 tsp. baking soda
1 tsp. baking powder
1 1/2 tsp. pumpkin pie spice
2 ripe bananas (mashed)
6 oz. can frozen orange juice
2 eggs
1 c. raisins
Nuts (optional)

Sift all dry ingredients together and set aside. In a separate bowl mix all wet ingredients and mashed bananas. Mix wet and dry ingredients together and mix well, then fold in, nuts and raisins. Pour in a greased and floured loaf pan unless using a non-stick pan. Bake at 350 - 375 degrees for 30-45 minutes or when knife comes out clean.

DIABETIC CHOCOLATE CHIP COOKIES

1/2 c. butter
1/3 c. brown Sugar Twin
1 egg
1 1/2 tsp. vanilla extract
1 1/3 c. all purpose flour
2 tsp. baking powder
1/2 tsp. baking soda
1/2 tsp. salt

3/4 c. skim milk
1/2 c. semi-sweet chocolate chips

Cream butter, brown sugar twin, vanilla and egg together. Sift all dry ingredients together in a separate bowl. Add milk, dry ingredients and chocolate chips to creamed mixture. Drop onto cookie sheet. Bake at 325-350 degrees for 7- 10 min. or until lightly brown.

WACHY CHOCOLATE CAKE

1 1/2 c. cake flour
1/4 c. cocoa
2 tbsp. granulated sugar replacement
1 tsp. baking soda
1/2 tsp. salt
1 c. water
1 tbsp. white vinegar
1/4 c. safflower or corn oil
1 tsp. vanilla extract
1 egg

Sift all dry ingredients together and set aside. In a separate bowl mix all wet ingredients. Mix wet and dry ingredients together and mix well. Pour in a greased and floured cake pan unless using a non-stick pan. Bake at 350 degrees for 25 –30 minutes or until cake springs back when lightly touched in the middle.

APPLE PIE, SUGARLESS

12 oz. can concentrated apple juice
3 tbsp. cornstarch
1 tsp. ground cinnamon
1/8 tsp. salt
9 inch unbaked pie shell
5 sweet tasting apples, sliced

Mix all ingredients and bring to a boil. When mixture starts to thicken remove from heat. Pour into pie crust. Bake at 350-375 degrees or until golden brown.

APPLESAUCE COOKIES

1/2 c. all purpose flour
1 tsp. ground cinnamon
1/2 tsp. baking soda
1/4 tsp. allspice
1/2 c. quick rolled oats
1/2 c. raisins
Nutmeats (Optional)
1/2 c. unsweetened applesauce
1 egg, beaten
1/4 c. shortening
2 tsp. vanilla extract
1/4 tsp. orange flavoring (optional)

Sift all dry ingredients (including oats) together in a separate bowl. In a separate bowl mix applesauce, eggs, vanilla, orange flavoring (optional) dry ingredients and nuts. Drop onto cookie sheet. Bake at 325-350 degrees for 7- 10 min. or until lightly brown.

DIABETIC OATMEAL COOKIES

3/4 c. vegetable shortening
1/2 c. Brown Sugar Twin
1/2 c. white Sugar Twin
1 egg
1/4 c. water
1 tsp. vanilla extract
1 c. all purpose flour
1 tsp. salt
1/2 tsp. baking soda
1 c. raisins
3 c. rolled oats, quick cooking or regular

Cream shortening,sugars, vanilla and egg together. Sift all dry ingredients together in a separate bowl. Add water, dry ingredients, raisins and oats to creamed mixture. Drop onto cookie sheet. Bake at 325-350 degrees for 7- 10 min. or until lightly brown

----

HELEN'S LOW - CAL PECAN PIE

9 inch unbaked pie shell
3/4 c. egg substitute
3 tbsp. all purpose flour
1/3 c. plus 1 tbsp. plus 1 tsp. thawed frozen pineapple juice concentrate
1/4 c. sugar
1/4 c. dark corn syrup
2 tbsp. reduced calorie tub margarine, melted
1 1/2 tsp. vanilla extract
1/8 tsp. salt
3 1/2 oz. pecan halves

Mix all ingredients except flour and pecans and bring to a boil. Now add flour and pecans. When mixture starts to thicken remove from heat. Pour into pie crust. Bake at 350-375 degrees or until golden brown on edges.

SUGAR - FREE SPICE COOKIES

2 c. water
1 c. raisins
2 sticks margarine
1 c. prunes, chopped
1 c. dates, chopped
2 egg whites
2 tsp. soda
1/2 tsp. salt
2 tsp. vanilla
1/2 tsp. cinnamon
1/2 tsp. nutmeg
Dash cloves
2 1/3 c. flour, and maybe 1/4 more
1/2 - 1 c. nuts

Cream margarine, vanilla and egg whites together. Sift all dry ingredients together in a separate bowl. Add water, dry ingredients, raisins, dates, prunes and nuts to creamed mixture. Drop onto cookie sheet. Bake at 325-350 degrees for 7- 10 min. or until lightly brown

----

DIABETIC BARS

1 c. dates
1/2 c. prunes
1 c. water
1 stick margarine
2 eggs
1 tsp. soda
1 tsp. vanilla
1/4 tsp. salt
1 c. flour
1/2 c. chopped nuts

Cream margarine, vanilla and egg together. Sift all dry ingredients together in a separate bowl. Add water, dry ingredients, dates, prunes and nuts to creamed mixture. Spread in a cookie sheet pan. Bake at 325-350 degrees for 15-20 min. or until lightly brown

----

PICKLED FRENCH STYLE GREEN BEANS

1 can beans
1 tsp. pickling spice
2 tsp. artificial sweetener
1/3 c. vinegar

Steam beans 5 minutes or less and strain. Mix rest of ingredients and bring to a boil. Strain to rid of spices. If needed you can add vinegar or sweetener to taste. Pour over beans and let stand overnight.

ALOHA SEAFOOD DISH

2 lbs. fish fillets
1/2 c. pineapple juice
1/4 c. steak sauce
1 tsp. salt
Dash of pepper

Place fish in single layer in shallow baking dish. Combine remaining ingredients and pour over fish. Let stand 30 minutes, turn once. Remove fish, reserving sauce for basting. Place fish on Pam sprayed broiler pan. Broil about 4 minutes, brushing with sauce. Turn carefully and brush with sauce. Broil until fish flakes when tested with fork. Garnish with lime wedges or pineapple if desired.

APPLE MAGIC

2 med. apples, pared, cored, coarsely chopped
1 1/2 tsp. cinnamon
Artificial sweetener to equal 5 tsp. sugar
2 envelopes (2 T) unflavored gelatin
10 to 12 fluid ounces lemon-flavored dietetic soda

Preheat oven to 350 degrees. In a deep, narrow, oblong pan arrange apples in layers. Combine 1 teaspoon cinnamon with sweetener to equal 1 teaspoon sugar. Sprinkle some of this mixture over each layer of apples. Sprinkle gelatin over 10 fluid ounces soda to soften. Add remaining sweetener and cinnamon; stir until dissolved. Pour mixture over apples; add remaining soda to cover apples. Bake at 350 degrees for 1 hour or until cooked throughout. While hot, refrigerate immediately, 4 to 6 hours or until set. Makes 2 servings.

APPLE TURNOVER

1 apple, peeled, cored and sliced
1 tsp. lemon juice
1 tbsp. water
1 slice white bread
1/4 tsp. cinnamon
Artificial sweetener to equal 2 tsp. sugar

Cook sweetener, cinnamon, water, and lemon juice with apple. Cook until tender. Cool. Remove crust from bread. Roll thin. Place apple mixture on 1/2 bread. Fold diagonally. Moisten edges and press together with fork. Bake at 425 degrees slower until crisp.

APPLE/PEAR TUNA SALAD

1 med. apple or pear
1 (3 oz.) water packed tuna
2 tbsp. diced green pepper
1 tbsp. lo-cal French or Italian dressing
2 tsp. lemon juice
Pinch of artificial sweetener
Lettuce cup

Dice pear. Toss with tuna and green pepper. Combine dressing, lemon juice, and sugar substitute. Pour over salad and toss. Spoon into lettuce cup.

APRICOT UP-SIDE DOWN CAKE

12 frozen apricot halves, thawed
1/2 tsp. lemon juice
1/2 tsp. brown sugar replacement
1/4 tsp. cinnamon
2 slices white bread crumbs
1 tsp. baking powder
Dash of salt
2 eggs, separated
1/3 c. granulated sugar replacement
3 tbsp. hot water
1/2 tsp. vanilla

Preheat oven to 350 degrees. Combine apricots, lemon juice, brown sugar, and cinnamon. Spread on bottom of non-stick small baking dish. Combine crumbs, baking powder, and salt. Beat egg yolks. Gradually beat in sugar until yolks are thick and lemon colored. Beat in water, bread crumb mixture and extract. Beat egg whites with a pinch of salt until stiff, not dry. Fold into egg mixture. Spoon over apricots. Bake for 25 minutes or until cooked throughout. 2 servings.

BAKED APPLES

Apples
Cinnamon
Artificial sweetener
Non-sugar black cherry soda

Wash and core apples. Slit and peel 1/3 of the way down. Place apples in oven- proof dish and pour soda over them. Sprinkle with cinnamon and sweetener. Bake at 375 degrees until apples are tender.

BAKED BEANS

2 (16 oz.) cans French style beans
1 tbsp. dehydrated onion flakes
1 c. tomato juice
2 tsp. Worcestershire sauce
1 tsp. dry mustard
Artificial sweetener to equal 12 tsp. sugar

Drain beans and empty into bowl. Add remaining ingredients. Mix lightly and turn into baking dish. Bake at 350 degrees for 45 minutes.

BAKED CHICKEN WITH APPLES

2 1/2 to 3 lb. chicken, cut up
1/2 tsp. salt
1/4 tsp. pepper
1 chicken bouillon cube
1/2 c. boiling water
1/2 c. apple juice
2 c. sliced fresh green beans, French style
1 c. diced peeled apples
1 tbsp. flour

1 tsp. ground cinnamon
1 oz. bread

Sprinkle both sides of chicken with salt and pepper. Place chicken on a rack in a shallow open roasting pan. Bake in hot oven (450 degrees) until browned, about 20 minutes. Reduce oven temperature to 350 degrees. Remove chicken and rack; pour off any fat from pan. Return chicken to pan. Dissolve bouillon in boiling water. Pour over chicken along with apple juice. Stir in green beans. Cover and bake 25 minutes. Stir in apple. Cover and bake 10 minutes longer. Meanwhile, in small saucepan mix flour with cinnamon. Blend with 1 tablespoon of cold water. Stir in hot pan liquid. Cook and stir until mixture boils and thickens slightly. Serve with chicken and vegetables.

BANANA CREAM PIE

2 c. skim milk
4 eggs, separated
4 packs artificial sweetener
1 tsp. banana extract
1 banana, sliced
2 packets unflavored gelatin
1 tsp. vanilla

Sprinkle gelatin in 3/4 cup cold milk. Heat remaining milk. Add gelatin mixture and stir over low heat until dissolved. Beat egg yolks, add to hot mixture stirring constantly. When mixture thickens, add sweetener. Remove from stove. Add vanilla and banana flavoring. Pour half of filling in 8 inch pie plate. Place sliced bananas on top. Cover with rest of filling. Meringue: Beat egg whites until frothy. Add 1/2 teaspoon cream of tartar, 1 teaspoon vanilla. Add 4 packs of artificial sweetener, 1/4 teaspoon nutmeg and beat. Beat until stiff. Pile on top of banana filling. Put under broiler 1 to 2 minutes until golden brown. Refrigerate 4 hours before serving.

BAR-B-Q MEATBALLS

1 lb. ground chuck
1/2 c. liquid skimmed milk

1 med. onion, chopped
Salt & pepper to taste
1/2 c. diet catsup
1 tbsp. minced green peppers
1 tsp. prepared mustard
1 tbsp. vinegar
1 tbsp. minced onion
1 1/2 tbsp. Worcestershire sauce
2 packs Sweet & Low

Mix chuck, milk, onion, salt & pepper. Make into balls. Broil until brown (approximately 15 minutes). Sauce: Mix catsup, green pepper, mustard, and vinegar. Add minced onion, Worcestershire sauce, & Sweet'N Low. Pour over meat balls. Cook covered for 15 minutes at 400 degrees.

BAR-B-Q SAUCE

1 can tomato juice
1 onion, chopped
1 tbsp. mustard
1 tsp. chili powder
1/4 c. vinegar
Garlic powder to taste
1/2 tsp. paprika
1 tsp. Worcestershire sauce
Sweetener, salt, & pepper to taste

Combine, bring to a boil then lower heat and simmer until thick as you desire.

BAR-B-QUE CHICKEN

Chicken, boiled, skinned, boned, & chopped
1 can tomato juice
1 onion, chopped
1 tbsp. mustard
1 tsp. chili powder
Sweetener to taste
1/4 c. vinegar

Dash of garlic powder
Pinch of oregano

Mix all ingredients, excluding chicken, to make the sauce. Mix chicken and as much sauce as you like. Simmer and eat on bread or without.

BROILED CHICKEN WITH GARLIC

2 1/2 lbs. chicken, quartered
6 cloves garlic
3/4 tsp. powdered rosemary
Salt & pepper to taste
Chicken bouillon

Rub chicken with 2 pressed garlic cloves, and rosemary. Also rub with salt and pepper. Let stand 30 minutes. Put chicken in broiler pan and coat top with bouillon. Sprinkle with 2 slivered garlic cloves. Add a little bouillon to pan. Broil turning when half done. Coat top sides with bouillon and 2 more slivered garlics. Baste with pan drippings.

BRUNSWICK STEW

3 oz. chicken breast
3 oz. ground chuck, cooked
12 oz. tomato juice
1/2 sm. onion or dehydrated
1 c. water
1 pkg. beef bouillon
1/2 tsp. red pepper
1/8 c. vinegar

Skin chicken and boil until tender. Broil beef until brown. Debone, chop, and blend chicken in blender. Cook tomato juice, water, and onion slowly (30 minutes). Add bouillon, pepper, meat, and vinegar. Add salt and pepper to taste. Cook very slow in a soup pot until thick or use a crockpot.

BUTTERMILK SHERBET

2 c. buttermilk
Sugar substitute equal to 1/2 c. sugar
1 egg white
1 1/2 tsp. vanilla
1/2 to 1 cup crushed pineapple

Combine and blend well all ingredients except pineapple. Pour into container. Add pineapple. Freeze. Stir occasionally until firm.

CABBAGE RELISH

5 lbs. cabbage
1 jar pimento
1/2 tsp. mustard seed
1 1/2 tsp. celery seed
4 tbsp. dehydrated onions
1 pt. white vinegar
1 tsp. salt
Artificial sweetener to equal 2 1/2 cups sugar
1/2 tsp. turmeric

Grate or chop cabbage and pimento.   Mix remaining ingredients and heat mixture. When it comes to a rolling boil, cool. Pour over cabbage mixture. Store in covered jars or container in refrigerator. Will keep several weeks. Taste better after it sets for a day.

CABBAGE ROLLS

6 lg. cabbage leaves
1/2 lb. ground chuck
1 tbsp. minced onion
1 egg
2 slices white bread
Salt & pepper to taste
Tomato sauce

Boil cabbage leaves in salt water for 5 minutes, set aside. Mix ground chuck, onion, salt, pepper, egg, and bread. Carefully spread cabbage leaf. Roll up small roll of beef mixture. Secure with toothpick. Place rolls in boiler. Pour tomato sauce plus a can of water over. Simmer about 45 minutes.

CABBAGE SALAD

3 c. shredded cabbage
1 tsp. salt
1 shredded turnip (2 oz.)
1 shredded carrot (2 oz.)
1 chopped green pepper
1/4 tsp. dill seed

Cover cabbage with salt. Let stand for 45 minutes. Wash and dry thoroughly. Drain and squeeze all water out. Toss with other ingredients. Moisten with low-cal dressing.

CABBAGE SURPRISE

3 c. chopped cabbage
8 oz. ground chuck (raw)
1 tbsp. chopped onion
5 oz. tomato juice
Salt & pepper to taste

Broil cabbage until tender, drain liquid and save. Cook beef in Pam sprayed skillet, drain. Drain meat on paper towels. Combine ingredients and cook on low heat for 30 to 35 minutes. If more soup is desired, add liquid from cabbage.

CABBAGE WITH TOMATOES

2 med. onions, sliced
Artificial sweetener to equal 1 tbsp. sugar

1 med. cabbage, shredded
1 tsp. salt
1/2 tsp. caraway seeds
1 to 2 tbsp. vinegar
1/2 c. water
3 lg. tomatoes, peeled and chopped
1 tbsp. flour
Bouillon

In deep saucepan, saute' onions in small amount of bouillon. Saute' until soft and golden. Sprinkle with sugar. Add cabbage, salt, caraway, vinegar, and water. Simmer, covered, over low heat for 30 minutes. Add tomatoes and simmer, covered for 15 minutes more. Mix flour with 2 to 3 tablespoons of pan liquid. Make a smooth paste. Stir into cabbage. Cook, uncovered, stirring constantly until mixture thickens.

CARROT AND ORANGE SALAD

1 1/2 c. water
4 oz. grated raw carrots
4 oz. unsweetened orange juice
1 tbsp. unflavored gelatin
1 tbsp. lemon juice
Artificial sweetener equal to 2 tsp. sugar
1/4 tsp. salt
Lettuce leaves

Soften gelatin in 1/4 cup cold water. Add salt, sweetener, and 1 1/4 cups hot water. Stir until dissolved. Add orange and lemon juice. Set aside to stiffen slightly. Add raw carrots to gelatin and pour into mold. Make sure mold has been rinsed in cold water. Chill. Unmold on lettuce leaves.

CELERY SALAD

4 c. slivered celery, sliced diagonally
2 heads Boston lettuce
1 (12 oz.) yogurt

1 1/2 tbsp. lemon juice
1 1/2 tbsp. DiJon mustard
4 tbsp. finely chopped parsley
Salt and pepper

Cover and cook celery in very small amount of boiling water. Cook for 3 minutes. Drain and cool. Arrange on lettuce cups. Mix yogurt, lemon juice, mustard, and parsley. Season to taste and pour dressing over celery.

CHEESE AND ONION CASSEROLE

8 oz. onions. sliced
4 oz. Swiss cheese, grated
4 eggs, slightly beaten
2 c. skim milk
2 tsp. salt
1 tsp. pepper
1 tsp. garlic powder
4 slices enriched white bread, crumbled, divided in half

Combine all ingredients except 1/2 of bread crumbs. Combine in casserole dish; mix well. Top casserole with remaining bread crumbs. Bake at 350 degrees for 25 minutes. Bake longer if needed until cooked throughout. Makes 4 servings.

CHEESE CAKE

2 eggs
1 lb. Farmer's cheese
1/4 c. buttermilk
1 1/2 tbsp. liquid artificial sweetener
1 tbsp. lemon juice
1 tsp. vanilla
6 oz. cottage cheese
1/3 c. buttermilk
1/2 tsp. cinnamon
1 pkg. artificial sweetener

Blend eggs, Farmer's cheese, 1/4 cup buttermilk, then add liquid sweetener, lemon juice, and vanilla. Pour into Pyrex dish and bake at 375 degrees for 15 minutes. Pour on cream topping and bake another 5 minutes. *TOPPING*: Blend cottage cheese, buttermilk, cinnamon. Add sweetener and mix well.

CHERRY BANANA DESSERT

2 c. cherry flavored sugar free beverage
1 envelope cherry flavored gelatin
1 sm. banana, peeled and sliced

Sprinkle gelatin over 1 cup of beverage. Heat remaining beverage to a boil. Combine with gelatin mixture. Stir until gelatin is dissolved. Refrigerate until thick. Add bananas and chill until firm.

BAKED CHICKEN DINNER

4 oz. chicken
1 egg
4 oz. cooked peas
1/3 c. dry milk
2 tbsp. dehydrated onion flakes
2 tbsp. green peppers, diced
2 tbsp. Worcestershire sauce
1/2 tsp. salt, seasoned
1/2 c. water
2 tbsp. pimento, chopped

Combine all ingredients. Bake at 350 degrees for 45 minutes.

CHICKEN LIVERS HAWAIIAN

1/4 c. liquid chicken bouillon
1/2 c. chopped celery
1/2 c. chopped onion
1/2 med. green pepper, sliced

12 oz. chicken livers
1 c. pineapple chunks
1 1/4 tsp. brown sugar substitute
1 tsp. salt
1 tbsp. cider vinegar
Bean sprouts

Cook celery, onion, and green pepper in Pam sprayed skillet. Cook over medium- high heat until crisp, about 5 minutes. Add chicken liver and cook 10 minutes. Add chicken liver and cook 10 minutes. Stir frequently. Add pineapple. Dissolve salt, sugar, and vinegar with 1/2 cup water. Add to skillet. Serve on cooked hot bean sprouts.

CHICKEN LOAF

4 oz. chopped raw carrots
1 c. chopped raw celery
1 tbsp. dehydrated onions
1 sm. can pimento, chopped
4 tbsp. diet mayonnaise
1 1/2 c. water
2 pkg. or cubes chicken bouillon
3 envelopes unflavored gelatin
1 tsp. garlic salt
2 tbsp. mustard
1 tsp. lemon pepper
1 tsp. salt
1/2 tsp. pepper
16 oz. cooked, chopped chicken

Mix all ingredients except bouillon, water and gelatin. Dissolve bouillon in 1 cup water. Dissolve gelatin in remaining 1/2 cup water. Add gelatin to boiling bouillon. Add to mixture. Pour into loaf pan. Refrigerate. Unmold, slice and serve.

CHICKEN SALAD

12 oz. sliced chicken
1/2 c. chopped celery
1/4 c. shredded carrots

1/4 c. lo-calorie salad dressing or mayonnaise
1 1/2 tsp. lime juice
Salt & pepper to taste

Combine chicken celery, and carrots. Stir dressing, juice, salt and pepper. Pour over chicken mixture, tossing to coat well.

CHICKEN STEW

4 chicken breasts, stewed
1 (6 oz.) can mushrooms
1/2 med. head cabbage, chopped
2 med. onions, chopped
Salt, pepper and garlic to taste
1 (12 oz.) tomato juice

To stew chicken, cover with water and pressure 15 minutes. Remove chicken from water, add mushrooms, cabbage and onions. Add salt, pepper, and garlic to taste. Add tomato juice and chopped chicken. Simmer for about 1 hour.

CHOCOLATE BAR

1/2 c. crushed pineapple, in own juice, drained
1 envelope ALBA 77

Mix ingredients together. Make a tin foil pan the size of a large chocolate bar. Pour ingredients into pan and freeze. When frozen, break into chunks.

CHOCOLATE CREAM ROLL

1 pkg. chocolate ALBA
2 eggs
1/2 tsp. cream of tartar
1 1/2 tsp. vanilla
1 pkg. Sweet'N Low
1/2 c. fruit juice

1 envelope unflavored gelatin
1/2 c. evaporated skim milk
2 tbsp. lemon juice
1 tsp. vanilla

Blend ALBA, eggs, cream of tartar, and baking soda. Add 1 1/2 teaspoon vanilla and Sweet'N Low. Blend in blender. Blend until smooth. Pour onto wax paper lined small cookie sheet. Bake at 350 degrees for 15 to 20 minutes. Cool. Place on a slightly damp dish towel. Carefully peel away wax paper. Cool. Spread with cream filling and roll up "Jelly-roll" style. Place the roll in freezer for storage. Remove from freezer a few minutes before serving time. Slice. *CREAM FILLING*: Mix fruit juice, gelatin, and milk. Add lemon juice, add 1 teaspoon vanilla.

CHOCOLATE PUDDING

1/3 c. chocolate Alba skimmed milk
1 egg
3/4 c. water
Vanilla to taste
Tart shells

Mix ingredients. Cook until thick. Serve in tart shells.

CHRISTMAS COLE SLAW

1/2 head green cabbage
1/4 head purpose cabbage
1/3 c. chopped onions
1/3 c. chopped green peppers
1/2 c. diet mayonnaise
1 tsp. salt
2 tsp. artificial sweetener
1/4 tsp. pepper
1 tsp. vinegar
1 tsp. lemon juice

Shred cabbage, chop onions and peppers. Mix with other ingredients.

CRANBERRY GELATIN

4 c. fresh cranberries
1/4 c. cold water
20 packs Sweet'N Low
1 tsp. vanilla extract
1 1/2 c. water
1 envelope unflavored gelatin

Combine berries, 1 1/2 cups water, vanilla, and sweetener. Combine in large saucepan. Bring to a boil. Simmer 10 minutes or until all berries pop. Sprinkle gelatin on 1/4 cup water to soften. Dissolve in hot cranberry mixture. Pour into mold and chill until set.

CREAMED SAUCE

1 box frozen cauliflower or fresh
1 (4 oz.) can stem and pieces of mushrooms
1/2 tsp. onion flakes
1/2 tsp. garlic powder
Salt & pepper to taste

Cook cauliflower in water as directed. Put in blender, using water it's cooked in. Add mushrooms using water they are packed in. Add onion flakes, garlic powder, salt and pepper. Blend until smooth.

CREAMY CHOCOLATE FUDGE

4 tbsp. diet butter
1/4 c. brown sugar replacement
1/4 tsp. instant coffee
1 envelope and 1/2 tsp. unflavored gelatin
1/4 c. cream flavored diet soda
2/3 c. nonfat dry milk
1 1/3 c. Ricotta cheese
1 tbsp. chocolate extract
1/2 tsp. vanilla
2 tsp. artificial sweetener (liquid)

1/2 tsp. brown food coloring
2 pkg. W.W. dried apples

Place margarine in a small pan over hot water to melt. Sift brown sugar and coffee very slowly into margarine. Stir constantly. Soften gelatin in soda. Add nonfat dry milk. Add a few drops more of soda if needed. The mixture needs to be paste like. Combine gelatin mixture with margarine mixture. Stir constantly over hot water until thoroughly blended. Combine cheese, extracts, sweetener, and food coloring. Mix well. Fold gelatin-margarine mixture into Ricotta mixture. Pour into 8 x 8 x 2 inch pan. Refrigerate 2 hours. Freeze for firmer fudge. 20 squares.

CRUNCHY HAMBURGERS

1 lb. ground chuck
1 (16 oz.) can bean sprouts, drained
1 tbsp. Worcestershire sauce
1 tsp. salt
1 tsp. ginger
1/2 tsp. garlic
1/4 tsp. pepper

Combine all ingredients. Divide mixture into 4 equal portions. Broil on rack until cooled.

DELICIOUS SALMON

6 oz. salmon
1 tbsp. chopped green pepper
1/4 tsp. onion flakes
1/4 tsp. horseradish
1 to 2 tbsp. diet French dressing
3 oz. Swiss cheese
6 slices tomatoes

Mix first 5 ingredients well and divide into thirds. Spread on 3 slices of toast. Add 1 ounce cheese and two slices of tomato. Place under broiler until cheese bubbles.

DEVILED FISH BROIL

1 tsp. dehydrated onion flakes
1/4 tsp. Red Hot sauce
1/2 tsp. Worcestershire sauce
1/2 tsp. soy sauce
8 oz. uncooked fish fillet
1 tbsp. prepared mustard
1/2 tsp. parsley, fresh, minced

Combine all ingredients except fish. Mix well. Brush on both sides of fish. Broil until fish flakes easily with fork.

DIET PIZZA

1 oz. bread
2 oz. cheese
1/4 c. mushrooms, sliced
Pinch of garlic powder
Pinch of oregano
Tomato sauce or catsup (optional)

Put mushrooms on toast and cover with cheese. Sprinkle with seasonings. Broil in oven until cheese is hot and bubbly.

DIETER'S DIP

1 (8 oz.) cottage cheese
1 (6 to 7 oz.) white tuna, packed in water
3 tbsp. chopped pimento
2 tsp. grated onion
Salt & pepper to taste

Blend cottage cheese until smooth and soft. Use blender or electric mixer. Drain and flake tuna. Combine with cottage cheese and seasonings.

DIETER'S DRESSING

1 (10.5 oz.) can tomato soup, undiluted
1/2 c. tarragon vinegar
1 celery stalk, cut up
1 clove garlic
1 tsp. paprika
1 med. dill pickle
6 sprigs parsley
1 tbsp. Worcestershire sauce
1 tsp. prepared mustard

Place all ingredients in a blender in order listed. Cover and run on high speed until vegetables are chopped.

DILLY TUNA SALAD

1 (20 oz.) can pineapple chunks
1 (6 oz.) can tuna, drained
1 c. cucumbers, sliced
1/3 c. imitation mayonnaise
1/2 tsp. seasoned salt
1/4 tsp. dill seed

Drain pineapple, reserving 2 tablespoons of juice. Mix all ingredients except dill seed. Line salad bowl with crisp salad greens. Add above mixed ingredients. Sprinkle with dill seed.

DIPPIN PEAS SALAD

1 med. pear
1/2 c. cottage cheese
1 tsp. orange juice concentrate, thawed
1 to 2 tbsp. skim milk

Cut pear into wedges. Place cottage cheese and orange juice in blender. Blend until smooth, adding milk as needed. Mixture should be very thick. Pour into small dish. Use pear wedges to scoop up cottage cheese mixture. Makes 1 salad.

EGG SALAD

3 hard boiled eggs
3 oz. cottage cheese
1 tsp. mustard
1 tbsp. chopped onion
1 tbsp. dill cubes
Crazy salt
Pepper
Finely chopped celery

Finely chop eggs. Mix all together. Makes lunch for two. Good on sandwich with tomato. Vary seasoning to suit your taste.

FRUIT 'N BREAD PUDDING

3 slices enriched white bread
1 1/2 med. bananas, peeled and sliced
1/2 c. sliced peaches with juice
1/2 c. cranberries
1/2 c. brown sugar replacement
1/2 tsp. ground cinnamon
1/3 c. water
1/2 tsp. banana extract
1/2 tsp. brandy extract
Grated nutmeg (optional)

On baking sheet toast bread at 325 degrees until dry. Cut toast into cubes. Combine toast cubes and fruits. Dissolve brown sugar and cinnamon in water. Add extracts. Pour over fruit mixture, turn with spatula until well coated. Let stand 5 minutes. Turn again, scraping down sides of bowl. Place mixture in one-quart size oven-proof casserole. Bake uncovered for 30 minutes. Serve warm with dusting of grated nutmeg. Makes 3 servings.

FRUITED CHICKEN SALAD

3 oz. blended cottage cheese
2 tbsp. skim milk
1 tbsp. cider vinegar
2 tsp. grated onion
1 tsp. salt
1 med. green pear, cubed
1 med. apple, cubed
1 c. chopped celery
Lettuce leaves

Mix celery, apple, pear, chicken, and salt until smooth. Add onion, vinegar, milk, and cheese and toss. Serve on lettuce leaves. Makes 3 sandwiches.

HERB SEASONED BROCCOLI

1/2 c. water
1 pkg. instant chicken broth and seasoning mix
2 c. broccoli spears
1/2 tsp. marjoram
1/2 tsp. basil
1/4 tsp. onion powder
Dash of nutmeg
1 tbsp. margarine
2 tsp. lemon juice

Combine water and broth mixture. Add broccoli, sprinkle with seasonings. Cover, bring to boil, simmer 6 minutes until tender. Drain. Divide on plates. Top with margarine and lemon juice. 2 servings.

HERBED FISH FILLETS

1 lb. fillets
1/2 tsp. salt
Dash of garlic powder
1/4 oz. drained chopped mushrooms
1/8 tsp. ground thyme
1/2 tsp. onion powder
Dash of black pepper
1/2 tsp. dried parsley
1 tbsp. nonfat dry milk
1 tbsp. water
1/2 tsp. lemon juice

Sprinkle fish with salt and garlic powder. Mix remaining ingredients and spread over fish. Bake at 350 degrees for 20 minutes, until fish flakes with fork.

HOT OPEN FACED BEEF SANDWICH

1 tbsp. bouillon liquid
1 lb. lean ground beef
1 c. chopped green pepper
1 c. chopped onion
1 c. diet catsup
2 tbsp. prepared mustard
Artificial sweetener to equal 1 tsp. sugar
1 tbsp. vinegar
Toasted bread

Brown beef in bouillon. Meanwhile, prepare the vegetable mixture. Combine remaining ingredients. May prepare ahead to allow seasonings to blend. Add vegetable mixture to beef. Turn heat on low and simmer covered for 30 minutes. Toast bread and spoon mixture over.

IMITATION BAKED POTATOES

1 (oz.) pkg. frozen cauliflower
1 packet instant chicken bouillon

1 tsp. fresh chopped parsley
1 tbsp. skim milk
1 c. water

Dissolve bouillon in water, add cauliflower, and cook. Place in blender with other ingredients. Do not over blend.

LEMON--PINEAPPLE MOLD

1 envelope lemon gelatin
1 envelope lime gelatin
1 c. buttermilk
1 c. cottage cheese
1 1/2 c. boiling water
1 1/2 c. crushed pineapple

Dissolve gelatin in boiling water. Mix cheese and buttermilk in blender until smooth. Pour into gelatin mixture. Add crushed pineapple.   Let set in refrigerator until firm.

MARY JO'S CONGEALED SALAD

2 envelopes unflavored gelatin
1 grapefruit, peeled and sectioned
1 c. boiling water
1 c. diet ginger ale
1/2 c. lemon juice
2 envelopes Sweet'N Low
4 tsp. vinegar
1/2 tsp. salt
2 c. shredded cabbage

Soften gelatin in lemon juice. Add boiling water stirring to dissolve gelatin. Add diet ginger ale, Sweet'N Low, vinegar and salt. Let chill. When it begins to thicken, fold in grapefruit and cabbage.

MEAT LOAF

1 lb. ground chuck
1 c. evaporated skimmed milk
1 tbsp. dehydrated onion flakes
1/2 tsp. salt
1/4 tsp. pepper
1/4 tsp. dry mustard
1/4 tsp. sage
1/8 tsp. garlic salt
1/2 c. chopped celery
1 tbsp. Worcestershire sauce

Combine all ingredients and shape into a loaf. Bake on rack at 350 degrees for 1 to 1 1/2 hours.

MEXICAN SUPPER

8 oz. ground hamburger (or veal)
1/3 c. chopped green pepper
1/4 head cabbage
1/2 c. onion
1 c. tomato juice
Salt & pepper to taste
1 tsp. chili powder

Cook meat and green pepper in skillet. In blender, blend cabbage and onion. Drain cabbage mixture. In saucepan, put tomato juice, cabbage and veal mixtures. Add salt and pepper to taste. Add chili powder. Cook until cabbage is done.

MOCK FRUIT CAKE

1/3 c. instant non-fat milk
1/4 c. chilled orange juice
1/2 apple, cored and chopped
3/4 c. red currants
2 tsp. lemon juice
1/4 tsp. cinnamon

1/8 tsp. maple extract
1/8 tsp. vanilla
Artificial sweetener to equal 6 tsp. sugar
2 oz. bread, toasted and grated

Preheat oven to 350 degrees. Combine milk and orange juice in large bowl. Whip until stiff by hand or mixer. Fold in remaining ingredients. Line loaf pan with wax paper. Pour ingredients into pan and bake 1 hour. Remove and cool thoroughly. Divide in half.

NEXT--DAY TURKEY AND RICE

1 egg, slightly beaten
1/2 c. cooked, enriched rice
2 oz. cooked turkey
1/2 med. green pepper, chopped
1 oz. onion, chopped
3/4 tsp. monosodium glutamate (optional)
1/4 tsp. soy sauce
Pinch garlic salt

Cook egg in non-stick skillet over medium heat. Cook until cooked throughout. Cut in bite-size pieces. Add all remaining ingredients; mix well. Cook until heated throughout. Makes 1 serving.

ONION DIP

6 oz. cottage cheese
2 1/2 tbsp. lemon juice
2 tbsp. buttermilk
Dash of onion flakes
1/2 tsp. garlic salt
Cake coloring for looks

Blend until creamy. Serve with celery sticks or raw cauliflower.

ONION FRIED CHICKEN

1 broiler (2 1/2 to 3 lbs. cut up)
1 tsp. salt
1/2 tsp. pepper
2 onions, peeled and sliced
1/2 c. water

Skin chicken. Place chicken in non-stick pan. Sprinkle with salt and pepper, and place onion on top. Cover, cook on low heat for 30 minutes. Tilt lid so liquid will evaporate. Continue cooking for 20 minutes or until tender. Place chicken on platter. Return onions, add water, cook until thickened.

ORIENTAL PORK BAR--B--QUE

2 lbs. fresh center slice ham
6 tbsp. soy sauce
1/2 tsp. garlic powder
2 tsp. sherry flavoring
1/2 c. tomato sauce
1/4 c water

Trim fat away. Mix soy sauce, garlic, sherry, and tomato sauce. Pour over meat in flat pan. Let stand, covered, in refrigerator for 3 hours. Drain off marinade and pour into small pan. Add water and heat. Put meat under broiler or grill. Cook until browned. Serve hot Bar-B-Q sauce with meat.

ORIENTAL VEGETABLES

Fresh broccoli
Yellow squash
Zucchini squash
Onions
Bell pepper
Ginger
Garlic powder
Soy sauce

Mushrooms (optional)
Egg plant (optional)

Spray Teflon pan with Pam. Cover and stir fry a few minutes. Add soy sauce, lower heat and simmer for about 20 minutes.

OUR "MOUSSAKA"

1 c. eggplant, peeled and sliced very thin
1/2 tsp. salt
1/2 tsp. pepper
1/4 tsp. oregano
6 oz. ground beef, broiled and crumbled
1 med. tomato, sliced
1 tbsp. vegetable oil
1 slice enriched white bread, crumbled

Place eggplant flat on baking sheet. Sprinkle with salt, pepper and oregano. Bake at 350 degrees for 10 minutes, turning once. Place half of meat in baking dish. Spread half of eggplant on meat. Place half of tomato on eggplant. Repeat. Sprinkle oil on top. Sprinkle bread crumbs over casserole. Cover. Bake for 15 minutes or until heated throughout.

PARMESAN CAULIFLOWER

1 head cauliflower
Dash of Parmesan cheese

Cook cauliflower in boiling water about 15 minutes. Remove from water and drain. Divide into flowerets. Top with Parmesan cheese.

PICKLED BANANA PEPPERS

1/2 c. water
1 c. vinegar
Artificial sweetener to = 1 cup sugar

Mix together and bring to a boil. Pour over pepper rings packed in jar. Approximately 1 quart.

PICKLED OKRA

Garlic, 1 clove for each jar
Hot pepper, 1 for each jar
Dill seed, 1 tsp. for each jar
1 qt. white vinegar or apple cider
1 c. water
1/2 c. salt

Place garlic and pepper in bottom of hot pint jars. Pack firmly with clean young okra pods. Stem end must be open. Add dill seed. After packing jars, bring water, vinegar, and salt to boil. Simmer about 5 minutes and pour while hot over okra. Seal immediately. Set 8 weeks.

PINEAPPLE PORK CHOPS

6 pork chops
6 pineapple rings (canned in own juice)
1/2 c. pineapple juice
1/4 tbsp. brown sugar substitute
1/4 tsp. cinnamon
Dash of rosemary leaves
1 c. celery, cut into strips
1 green pepper, cut into strips

Trim all fat from meat. Brown meat on both sides in Pam-sprayed skillet. Remove chops. Clean pan of all fat. In skillet, mix pineapple juice and sugar substitute. Add cinnamon and rosemary. Put chops in pan. Sprinkle with salt and pepper. Add celery and cover. Simmer about 30 minutes. Add green pepper strips. Place pineapple rings on each chop. Cover and cook about 10 minutes longer. Arrange chops on serving platter. Place pineapple and pepper strips on top. Spoon juice over. Garnish with parsley.

PINEAPPLE PUDDING

3/4 c. dry non-fat milk
1 egg
30 drops liquid sweetener
1 tsp. vanilla
1 sm. can crushed pineapple, drained but save juice

Add enough water to pineapple juice to make 1/2 cup. Mix all except pineapple and cook until almost thick. Add pineapple and continue to cook until thick.

POTATO SALAD

2 pkgs. cauliflower
1/2 c. chopped celery
2 tbsp. dill salad cubes
1 tbsp. chopped pimento
1 tbsp. chopped bell pepper
2 tbsp. mustard
1 tbsp. vinegar
2 tbsp. diet mayonnaise
Sweetener, salt and pepper to taste

Cook cauliflower. Mix all ingredients together. Better if you can let chill a few minutes before eating.

PUMPKIN BREAD

1/2 c. pumpkin
1 oz. bread
2/3 c. dry skim milk powder
2 eggs
3 packs artificial sweetener
1/2 tsp. baking soda
1/4 tsp. cream of tartar
1/2 tsp. cinnamon

1/4 tsp. nutmeg
1/4 tsp. ginger
1/8 tsp. cloves
1/2 tsp. grated orange rind

Mix all ingredients in bowl with electric mixer until smooth. Pour into Pam sprayed loaf pan. Bake at 350 degrees for 30 to 45 minutes.

ROAST BEEF SANDWICH

3 oz. roast beef, diced
2 tbsp. chopped celery
1/8 tsp. chopped chives
1/2 tbsp. lemon juice
1/2 med. tomato, chopped
1/2 tsp. salt
1/4 tsp. pepper
1 tsp. diet mayonnaise
2 slices thin bread
Lettuce

Combine all ingredients except bread and lettuce. Mix well. Spread on one slice of bread. Top with lettuce and remaining bread.

SALMON OR TUNA PUFFS

8 oz. salmon or tuna, drained
1 c. skim milk
1/2 c. mushrooms, sliced
1/4 c. green pepper or pimento, chopped
Salt and pepper to taste
2 eggs, separated

Combine fish, skim milk, mushrooms, and green pepper. Bake at 375 degrees. Meanwhile, beat egg whites with a dash of salt until stiff. Beat egg yolks, fold whites into yolks a little at a time. Pour over hot mixture and return to oven for another 20 minutes.

SHEPHERD'S PIE

6 oz. cooked roast beef, cubed
Butter salt
Pepper
1 tbsp. dehydrated onion
2 beef bouillon cubes
3 to 4 oz. mashed cauliflower

Dissolve bouillon in enough water to make a gravy. Put all in a small baking dish, cover with cauliflower. Bake at 350 degrees. Bake until thoroughly heated and cauliflower is browned.

SKILLET EGGS

1/4 c. tomato juice
1/8 tsp. pepper
2 eggs
1/4 tsp. salt
1/4 tsp. parsley flakes

In skillet, combine all ingredients except eggs. Stir over moderate heat until mixture comes to a boil. Add eggs, one at a time. Cook over moderate heat basting with tomato juice. Baste until eggs are set. About 4 minutes.

SLUSHY

1 can sugar-free ginger ale
1/4 c. unsweetened pineapple juice
ice cubes Blend until slushy. May add rum extract.

SOUTHERN CELERY FISH SALAD

6 c. thinly sliced celery
1/2 c. sliced med. onion
1/2 c. diet mayonnaise
1 tsp. salt
1/4 tsp. pepper
2 lbs. fillet of sole or flounder, cooked, chunked, and chilled
1 1/2 c. orange sections

Combine all ingredients except fish and orange. Mix well. Add fish and orange, toss lightly. Serve on lettuce leaves. Garnish with tomato wedges and radish roses if desired.

SPAGHETTI

12 oz. tomato juice
1 lg. can mushrooms, stems and pieces
Salt to taste
Garlic to taste
Oregano to taste
Dehydrated onion flakes
1 lg. green pepper, diced
2 cans bean sprouts

Cook all ingredients in covered saucepan. Cook until mixture thickens. Add bean sprouts; simmer 10 minutes. Sauce will usually taste better after sitting over night in refrigerator.

SPANISH STRING BEANS

1 sm. jar pimento
1/4 tsp. onion flakes
2 tbsp. skim milk solids
1/2 c. chicken bouillon
1 (9 oz.) pkg. frozen French style green beans

Simmer pimentos, onion flakes and skim milk. Simmer in chicken bouillon for 10 minutes. Add frozen beans, cover and cook until beans are done. Do not over cook beans.

SPICY APPLE TWIST

1 sm. apple
2 thin slices white bread
Cinnamon and Sweet'N Low mixture

Peel, core and cut apple in quarters. Roll bread very thin. Cut off crusts. Sprinkle bread with cinnamon and Sweet'N Low mixture. Cut each slice of bread in 4 strips. Put 2 strips together with a little water. Now form 2 strips. Wrap brad around apple slice. Sprinkle generously with cinnamon and Sweet'N Low. Place in Pam sprayed pan. Bake at 450 degrees for 10 to 15 minutes.

SQUASH PICKLES

2 lb. squash
4 lg. onions
1/4 c. salt
2 c. vinegar
1 tsp. celery seed
1 tsp. turmeric
1 tsp. mustard seed
Diet sweetener to equal 2 cups sugar

Cover squash and onions and salt with cold water. Let set 2 hours. Drain. Mix all ingredients together and let set 2 hours longer. Bring to a boil for 5 minutes and pack in hot jars.

STRAWBERRY CHIFFON PIE

1 c. crushed pineapple, unsweetened
12 strawberries
1 pkg. O-Zenta strawberry gelatin
7 pkgs. artificial sweetener
1 c. evaporated skim milk, chilled
1 tbsp. lemon juice
1 1/2 tsp. vanilla
1 tsp. almond extract

Bring pineapple to boil. Stir in strawberries, gelatin, and sweetener. Stir until gelatin is dissolved. Whip milk and lemon juice in chilled bowl until frothy. Add extracts and beat until stiff. Add gelatin mixture slowly to whipped milk. Pile into 10 inch pie plate and refrigerate.   Garnish with additional strawberries.

STRAWBERRY FRUIT SQUARES

2 envelopes dietetic strawberry gelatin
1 c. boiling water
1 c. crushed pineapple, in own juice
1 ripe banana, finely diced
6 oz. plain yogurt
1 envelope Sweet'N Low

Dissolve gelatin in boiling water. Add juice drained from pineapple with cold water. Enough cold water to equal 1 cup liquid. Add pineapple and banana. Pour 1/2 into 1 quart bowl. Chill until firm. Spread evenly with plain yogurt mixed with sugar substitute. Place bowl in freezer for 30 minutes until yogurt is firmer.   Pour remaining gelatin, very carefully, on top. Chill until firm. Cut in squares.

STRAWBERRY--PRAMGE DELIGHT

1/2 c. unsweetened orange juice
24 unsweetened strawberries
Artificial sweetener to equal 2 tsp. Sugar

Blend in blender and freeze until firm.

SWEET 'N SOUR CABBAGE

4 c. shredded cabbage
3 oz. ham
2 tbsp. artificial brown sugar
1 tbsp. flour
1/4 c. water
1/3 c. vinegar
1 sm. onion, sliced
2 cloves
Salt and pepper to taste

Cook cabbage in boiling salted water approximately 7 minutes. Add sugar and flour to small amount of bouillon; blend. Add the 1/4 cup water, vinegar, and seasonings. Cook until thick. Add onion, diced ham, and cabbage. Heat thoroughly.

SWEET AND SOUR CAULIFLOWER

1 c. fresh cauliflower, bite size pieces
1 c. boiling water
1/2 tsp. salt
1 tbsp. brown sugar replacement
2 tsp. lemon juice
1 tsp. margarine

Place cauliflower, water and salt in saucepan. Cook over medium heat covered. Cook for 10 minutes or until just barely tender. Drain. Combine brown sugar replacement, lemon juice and margarine. Combine in custard cup over hot water. When blended, pour over cauliflower.

TACOS

5 oz. raw ground veal (can also use lean beef)
1 tsp. chili powder
1 tsp. dehydrated onion
1/4 tsp. salt
1/4 tsp. onion powder
1/4 tsp. paprika

Dash Red Hot sauce
1 oz. bread (1 slice)
1/2 c. shredded lettuce
1 tbsp. pimento dressing
1 (7 oz.) jar pimento, drained
2 tbsp. vinegar
2 tbsp. prepared mustard
Artificial sweetener equal to 4 tsp. sugar

Brown meat in Pam sprayed skillet. Add seasonings and cook 5 minutes. Remove meat from skillet. Toast bread lightly. Spread meat mixture over 1/2 of the slice. Fold and hold in place with toothpick. Combine lettuce and pimento dressing. Cover taco. Makes 1 serving. Pimento Dressing: Combine pimento, vinegar and mustard. Add sweetener. Blend until smooth. Store in refrigerator and use as desired. Makes 1 cup.

THOUSAND ISLAND DRESSING

4 oz. tomato juice
2 tbsp. vinegar
1/4 c. finely chopped green pepper
1 tsp. Worcestershire sauce
1/2 tsp. salt
1/2 tsp. dry mustard
Garlic salt to taste
3 tbsp. finely diced dill pickle
3 tbsp. finely diced pimento
2 tsp. finely minced parsley
1/4 tsp. liquid sugar substitute

Blend and store in refrigerator. Use as needed.

TUNA A LA KING

1 (3 oz.) can tuna
2 oz. skimmed milk
Salt and pepper
1/2 sm. can mushrooms (stems and pieces)
Bread, toasted

Drain mushrooms and place into blender. Add milk and seasonings and puree'. Heat in saucepan with tuna. Pour over toast.

TUNA CASSEROLE

1 (6 oz.) drained tuna
2 oz. grated cheese
1 egg
1 c. asparagus
2 ribs celery, chopped

Combine all ingredients. Bake in lightly greased pan at 350 degrees until dry.

TUNA SALAD

2 oz. tuna, drained
2 tbsp. low-cal Thousand Island dressing
1 stalk celery, chopped
1 hard boiled egg
3 oz. cottage cheese

Mix all ingredients and serve on lettuce leaf or bread.

TURKEY AND POTATO SALAD

4 oz. cooked turkey or chicken, bite size pieces
1 (3 oz.) boiled potato, chopped
1 tbsp. mayonnaise
1 tsp. chopped pimento
1/2 tsp. dehydrated parsley flakes
1/2 tsp. nutmeg
1/2 tsp. sage
1/4 tsp. salt
Dash of pepper
Lettuce leaves

Combine all ingredients except lettuce; mix well. Chill. Serve on lettuce leaves. Makes 1 serving.

TURKEY CASSEROLE

1/2 c. cooked, enriched noodles
4 oz. cooked turkey, bite-size pieces
1/2 c. green beans, divided
1/4 c. canned, sliced mushrooms
1 oz. red onion, chopped
1 tsp. chopped pimento
1/4 tsp. nutmeg
1/4 tsp. salt
2 tbsp. skim milk

Combine noodles, turkey, 1/4 cup green beans, and mushrooms. Add onion, pimento, nutmeg and salt. Pour into baking dish. In blender, combine remaining green beans and milk. Mix until smooth. Add green bean sauce to casserole. Mix well. Bake at 350 degrees for 20 minutes. 1 serving.

VEAL STEW--PENDOUS

2 lb. veal, cut into cubes
12 oz. tomato juice
1 pkg. frozen peas
1 pkg. French style green beans
1 pkg. zucchini slices
1 tbsp. minced onions
1 tbsp. granulated brown sugar (twin)
Garlic powder, salt and pepper to taste
1/2 tsp. cinnamon

Brown meat in lightly greased pan. Combine with tomato juice, onion, salt, and pepper. Simmer until meat is tender or pressure cook about 10 minutes. Add frozen vegetables, and simmer until vegetables are done.   Add garlic powder, brown sugar substitute, and cinnamon. Serves 6.

VELVIA'S MIXED SALAD

1/2 head lettuce, chopped
2 slices pineapple, in own juice
4 oz. diced chicken
1 boiled egg
4 radish, diced
1/2 med. onion, diced
1 tbsp. diet mayonnaise

Combine all ingredients and mix well.

ZIPPY TOMATO RELISH

12 ripe tomatoes, chopped in large pieces
2 big onions, chopped in large pieces
2 bell peppers or 5 sweet banana peppers, chopped in large pieces
2 c. vinegar
Artificial sweetener to equal 2 cups sugar
2 tbsp. salt

Mix all ingredients and simmer about 2 hours.

MACARONI AND CHEESE

1/2 c. non-fat skim milk
1 oz. cheese
1 oz. bread
Salt & pepper to taste
Dash of paprika
Dash of mustard
Dash of cayenne
1 egg, separated

Heat milk (do not boil), add cheese, bread, and seasonings. As soon as cheese melts, remove from heat. Add beaten egg yolks. Beat whites stiff and fold in. Bake at 350 degrees for 25 minutes until brown.

COCKTAIL MEATBALLS

2 lbs. hamburger
1 med. onion, chopped
1 c. cracker crumbs
1/2 c. skim milk
2 eggs
Dash of garlic powder
Salt and pepper to taste

--SAUCE--
1 1/2 c. ketchup
1/3 c. vinegar
1/4 c. yellow mustard
Brown sugar substitute equivalent to 3/4 c. brown sugar

Mix ingredients together. Roll into walnut size balls and place in 9 x 13 inch baking dish. You should be able to place 6 balls width wise in baking dish and 10 balls lengthwise. Sauce: Mix in glass measuring cup. Pour over meatballs and bake in 350 degree oven for 1 hour. Makes about 60 meatballs.

LUNCHEON CASSEROLE

--WHITE SAUCE--
4 to 6 tbsp. flour
2 c. milk
1 lg. can tuna (crab, salmon, or 3 c. cooked chicken), diced
1 1/2 c. celery, chopped
1 lg. jar pimento
1/2 c. green pepper, chopped
1/2 c. sliced almonds
4 hard boiled eggs
1 tsp. salt
1 box fresh mushrooms
1/2 c. dry bread crumbs

Saute celery and peppers in ½ c. of margarine. Make white sauce. Layer fish or chicken, celery, pepper, pimento, nuts, eggs, and mushrooms. Pour white sauce over top of casserole. Top with bread crumbs. Bake in 350 degree oven for 50 minutes. Makes 10 generous servings.

REUBEN CASSEROLE

1 (16 oz.) pkg. sauerkraut from refrigerator section
2 c. shredded Swiss cheese
1/4 c. Thousand Island dressing
2 med. tomatoes, sliced
1/4 c. dried pumpernickel bread
   crumbs (2 or 3 slices)
1 (12 oz.) can corn beef, broken into sm. pieces
1/2 c. lite mayonnaise
1 tsp. Dutch mustard
2 tsp. melted margarine

Place sauerkraut in 1 1/2 quart casserole. Top with corned beef and then shredded cheese. Combine mayonnaise and Thousand Island. Spread over cheese. Top with tomatoes. Set aside. Microwave margarine 1 minute until melted. Stir bread crumbs into margarine. Sprinkle buttered crumbs over tomato slices. Microwave on roast to 12 to 14 minutes until heated through. Let stand 5 minutes before serving.

SWISS STEAK

1 1/2 lbs. lean round steak
2 tbsp. flour
1/2 tsp. seasoned salt
1/8 tsp. paprika
Vegetable cooking spray
1/2 c. beef broth
1/2 c. vegetable juice (V-8)
1/4 tsp. dried thyme
1 med. onion, sliced
2 carrots, cut into thin strips
2 stalks celery, cut into thin strips
1 lg. leek, cut into thin strips (optional)
1 tbsp. parsley

Cut steak into serving size pieces. Trim fat. Combine flour, salt, and paprika. Drench steak in flour mixture. Pound steak with mallet. Coat skillet with cooking spray. Put pan on medium heat until hot. Brown steak on both sides. Remove and drain on paper towel. Wipe pan drippings from skillet with paper towel. Combine broth, vegetable juice, and thyme in skillet. Bring to boil and return meat to skillet. Add onion. Cover; reduce heat and simmer for 1 hour. At end of hour, add celery, carrots, and leek. Simmer, uncovered, for 15 minutes until the vegetables are tender. Sprinkle with parsley. Makes 6 servings.

TURKEY STUFFED ZUCCHINI

4 med. zucchini, halved lengthwise
1 lb. ground turkey
1/4 c. onion, chopped
1 garlic clove, minced
1 tbsp. margarine
1 sm. tomato, chopped (1/2 c.)
1 tbsp. chopped parsley
1/2 tsp. salt
1/4 tsp. basil
1/8 tsp. pepper
1/2 c. crunchy nut (cereal nuggets or Grapenuts)
1 (8 oz.) container plain low-fat yogurt

Remove pulp from zucchini; chop and set aside. Parboil zucchini shells in boiling water to cover for 1 minute. Drain and place in shallow baking dish. Sautee turkey, onion, and garlic in margarine in skillet for 2 minutes. Add chopped pulp, tomato, parsley, salt, basil, and pepper.

Sautee about 5 minutes longer or until zucchini is tender. Add cereal and 1/2 cup of the yogurt. Spoon into shells. Bake at 350 degrees for 10 to 15 minutes or until shells are tender. Serve with remaining yogurt. Sprinkle with additional chopped parsley, if desired. Makes 4 servings.

LO - CAL EGGPLANT

1 eggplant
1 onion
Parmesan cheese
Salt
Pepper

Peel eggplant and dice into salted boiling water. Slice onion into the water too; cook about 20 minutes. Drain and toss with cheese, salt, and pepper to taste.

LOW CAL RHUBARB TORTE

1 c. flour
1/2 c. butter or oleo
5 tbsp. powdered sugar
1/8 tsp. salt
2 eggs
1 1/2 c. Sugar Twin
1/4 c. flour
3/4 tsp. baking powder
3 c. rhubarb

Crust: Mix 1 cup flour, butter, powdered sugar, and salt together. Pat into a 12 x 7 x 1/2 inch cake pan. Bake 10 minutes at 375 degrees. Remove from oven and cool slightly. *Filling:* Mix eggs, Sugar Twin, 1/4 cup flour, baking powder, and rhubarb together. Cover the crust with this mixture. Bake 35 to 40 minutes at 375 degrees.

COPPER PENNY CARROTS

2 lbs. carrots, cleaned and sliced thin
1 green pepper, thinly sliced
1 med. onion, thinly sliced
Salt and pepper as desired

--SAUCE--
1/4 c. salad oil
1 tsp. Worcestershire sauce

1 (10 oz.) can tomato soup, undiluted
1 tsp. yellow mustard
1/2 c. vinegar
20 packets Equal

Cook carrots in covered pan in 1/2 inch of water, 8 minutes after boiling has started (so carrots are tender but still crunchy). Rinse in cold water to stop cooking. In bowl, alternate layers of vegetables. Sauce: Bring sauce ingredients to a boil, stirring occasionally. Remove from heat.

Cool for a few minutes. Add 20 packets Equal. Put in blender and blend. Pour sauce over vegetables while still hot. Cool. Refrigerate at least 12 hours before serving. Will keep in refrigerator several weeks in a covered plastic container. To serve, use a slotted spoon.

SWEETLY POACHED PEARS

6 med. ripe pears (about 2 lbs.)
5 c. white, unsweetened grape juice
1/4 c. fresh lemon juice
1 vanilla bean, split lengthwise
1 inch whole cinnamon stick
1/4 c. golden raisins

Peel pears, leaving stems on. In a medium size pan, heat juices, vanilla bean, and cinnamon stick to a simmer. Add pears. Simmer 25 to 30 minutes, uncovered, turning pears occasionally, until tender when pierced with a knife. Remove pears with a slotted spoon. Reduce syrup 30 to 35 minutes to 1 1/2 cups. Strain.

Stir in raisins and cool syrup to room temperature. Serve pears in small glass compote bowls. Spoon raisins and syrup over and around pears. Serves 6. *Per serving: 187 calories, 48 gm carbohydrates, 1 gm protein, trace fat, 3 gm sodium. Exchanges: 3 fruit. Cholesterol: 9 mg per serving.*

CHOCOLATE CHEESECAKE

Margarine for pan
15 oz. part skim milk Ricotta cheese
1 1/2 c. (12 oz.) light cream cheese, softened
1 whole egg
2 egg whites
1 c. unsweetened apple juice concentrate
3 tbsp. unsweetened cocoa
1 tbsp. cornstarch
1 tbsp. sugar
1 tsp. vanilla extract
2 tsp. unsweetened cocoa (for topping)

Preheat oven to 350 degrees. Lightly grease bottom and sides of a 9 inch spring-form pan. Wrap outside of pan with aluminum foil. In the bowl of a food processor or blender, puree all ingredients until smooth. Do in 2 batches, if necessary.

With a rubber spatula, scrape mixture into prepared pan. Place on a baking sheet. Bake 45 minutes. Turn oven off. Leave in the oven with door closed for 1 hour. Remove and refrigerate. Before unmolding and serving, let stand at room temperature for 10 minutes. Sift 2 teaspoons unsweetened cocoa over the top.

Slice with a knife which has been warmed in hot water. Serves 12. Per serving: *167 calories, 16 gm carbohydrates, 8 gm protein, 8 gm fat, 220 mg sodium. Exchanges: 1 fruit, 1 medium fat meat, 1/2 fat. Cholesterol: 50 mg per serving.*

DIABETIC DATE NUT CAKE

1 1/2 stick margarine
2 tbsp. sweetener (or to taste - Iusually put in more)
1 c. chopped dates or raisins
1 1/2 c. unsweetened applesauce
1 c. pecans, chopped
1/2 tsp. cinnamon
1/2 tsp. cloves
1 tsp. vanilla
2 tsp. soda

2 c. plus 2 tbsp. all-purpose flour

Have margarine at room temperature. Mix margarine, applesauce, sweetening, sifted flour, soda, cloves, and cinnamon together. Put pecans, raisins, or dates in bowl and add a few spoons of the flour mixture; stir until the pecans and fruit are coated. Mix well and bake in tube pan. Line bottom of pan with wax paper. This cake tastes like fruit cake.

CARROT CAKE

Margarine and flour for pan
1 1/2 c. all-purpose flour
1/4 c. whole wheat flour
1 tsp. baking powder
1/2 tsp. baking soda
1/2 tsp. ground cinnamon
1/2 tsp. ground ginger
1/4 tsp. salt
1/2 c. vegetable oil
6 tbsp. sugar
2 eggs
1/4 c. unsweetened pineapple juice concentrate
1 tsp. vanilla extract
1 c. shredded carrots
1/2 c. golden raisins
1/2 c. unsweetened, crushed pineapple, drained

Preheat oven to 350 degrees. Grease and flour a 9 x 5 x 3 inch loaf pan. In bowl, toss flours, baking powder, baking soda, cinnamon, ginger, and salt. In a second bowl, stir oil, sugar, eggs, pineapple juice, and vanilla. Stir liquid into dry ingredients until smooth. Stir carrots, raisins, and pineapple. Scrape into prepared pan. Bake for 35 to 40 minutes until a pick inserted in the center of the cake comes out clean. Cool in pan on a rack for 1 hour. Unmold cake and ice with Cream Cheese Frosting. Cut into 1/2 inch slices to serve. Serves 18. *Per serving: 142 calories, 19 gm carbohydrates, 2 gm protein, 7 gm fat, 87 mg sodium. Exchanges: 1 starch, 1 fat. Cholesterol: 30 mg per serving.*

CREAM CHEESE FROSTING

8 oz. light cream cheese, room temperature
5 tbsp. unsweetened pineapple juice concentrate
1/2 tsp. vanilla extract
1/2 tsp. finely grated orange zest

In a bowl, whisk all ingredients together until smooth. Yield: About 1 1/4 cups. *Per serving: 46 calories, 3 gm carbohydrates, 2 gm protein, 3 gm fat. 96 mg sodium. Exchanges: 1 fat. Serving size: 1 1/2 tablespoons. Cholesterol: 10 mg per serving.*

DATE COFFEE CAKE

1/3 c. mashed banana, mash ripe banana with fork
1/2 c. margarine, softened
3 lg. eggs
1 tsp. vanilla extract
1 1/4 c. water
3 c. unbleached white flour
1 tsp. baking soda
2 tsp. baking powder
1 1/2 c. chopped dates

--TOPPING--
1/3 c. chopped dates
1/3 c. chopped walnuts
1/3 c. flaked coconut

Beat together mashed banana and margarine until creamy. Add eggs, vanilla, and water; beat. Measure in flour, baking soda, and baking powder. Beat well. Stir 1 1/2 cups chopped dates. Spoon batter into an oiled and floured 9 x 13 inch baking pan. Spread batter evenly in pan. Combine topping ingredients and sprinkle over batter. Bake in 350 degree oven for 20 to 25 minutes or until knife inserted comes out clean. Cool on a wire rack. Serves 10.

BLUEBERRY MUFFINS

1 c. all-purpose flour, sifted

1 1/2 tsp. baking powder
1/2 tsp. salt (optional)
1 1/2 tsp. or 2 pkgs. Equal
1/2 c. skim milk
1 egg or 1/4 c. Egg Beater
2 1/2 tbsp. melted shortening
1/3 c. fresh or frozen blueberries

Preheat oven to 425 degrees. Spray muffin tins with non-stick vegetable spray. Sift together flour, baking powder, and salt. Beat Equal and egg together. Add milk and melted shortening. Stir into the flour mixture. Stir in blueberries until just mixed. Batter will be slightly lumpy. Divide into tins. Bake 20 to 25 minutes or until done.

MICROWAVE BRAN MUFFINS

1 c. bran
1 c. buttermilk
1 banana, mashed well
1 egg
1/4 c. oil
1/4 c. honey
1 c. whole wheat flour
1 tsp. baking soda
Pinch of salt
2 tbsp. margarine
2 tbsp. honey

Mix first 9 ingredients together. Place in microwave muffin pan. Microwave 3 1/2 minutes. Mix last 2 ingredients together. Spoon on each muffin and return to microwave for 1 minute. Makes 12.

BANANA PECAN CREAM PIE

1 c. sugar free cookie crumbs
1/4 c. finely chopped pecans
2 tbsp. margarine, softened

--FILLING--
1 3/4 c. skim milk

1/4 c. unsweetened apple juice concentrate
1/4 c. cornstarch
4 tsp. sugar
1 tsp. vanilla extract
Pinch of salt
2 tbsp. margarine
2 med. bananas, sliced
1/4 c. sugar free cookie crumbs
1/4 c. chopped pecans

To make Crust: Blend cookie crumbs, pecans, and margarine in a bowl. Press into a 9 inch pie plate. Chill 30 minutes. To make Filling: In a saucepan, heat all filling ingredients, except margarine, to a boil over medium heat, whisking until smooth (about 10 minutes). Reduce heat and simmer for 1 minute. Scrape into a bowl. Whisk in remaining 2 tablespoons of margarine until smooth. Cover with plastic wrap and cool to room temperature. In prepared pie plate, arrange sliced bananas in 1 layer. Whisk cooled filling and pour evenly over bananas. Mix remaining cookie crumbs and pecans together and sprinkle over the filling. Chill for 1 hour before serving. Serves 8 to 12. *Per serving: 172 calories, 22 gm carbohydrate, 3 gm protein, 11 gm fat, 146 mg sodium. Exchanges: 1 starch, 1/2 fruit, 2 fat. Cholesterol: 0 mg per serving.*

DIABETIC KEY LIME PIE

1 (13 oz.) can evaporated skim milk
2 tsp. vanilla
2 envs. plain gelatin
1/3 c. lime juice, strain if fresh
1 c. boiling water
20 pkgs. Equal
Zest of 3 limes, grated rind
Green food coloring

Combine milk and vanilla. Freeze for 30 minutes. Combine gelatin and juice in a blender. Let set for 1 minute. Add boiling water and Equal; blend until smooth. Chill about 45 minutes. Put frozen milk into a small chilled bowl and whip frozen milk until stiff. Fold in lime zest. Slowly add the gelatin mixture to whipped milk. Spoon into 2 cooked pie shells or you may use a 9 x 13 inch baking dish. Garnish

with lime slices and zest. Makes 16 servings. See recipe for Diabetic
Pie Crust below

DIABETIC PIE CRUST

20 graham crackers, crushed
4 tbsp. oleo, melted
2 pkgs. Equal
1/4 lemon peel (optional)

Crush crackers and add Equal. Add oleo. Put in pie plates and pat
down. Put in refrigerator for 1 hour to chill. Makes 2 (9 inch) pie
crusts or 1 (9 x 13 inch) baking dish crust.

NO SUGAR CUSTARD PIE

1 lg. can evaporated milk
3 eggs
1 tbsp. cornstarch
15 packets Equal

Combine ingredients and beat lightly. Add ONE of the following: 2 c.
pears, grated and spices 2 lg. apples, grated and spices 2 c. peaches,
grated and spices 1 1/2 c. flake coconut and 1 tsp. vanilla 1 can
pumpkin and spices 2 c. drained and mashed, cooked butternut
squash and spices

--TOPPING FOR SQUASH AND PUMPKIN--
1/2 c. crushed cereal flakes
1/4 c. coconut
1/4 c. chopped pecans
1/2 stick butter

Pour pie ingredients into large unbaked pie shell. Bake on bottom rack
of oven at 350 degrees for 30 to 35 minutes. For Pumpkin or Squash
Topping: Mix together and sprinkle on top of pie. Bake on top rack
for last 10 minutes.

COCONUT SURPRISES

3 oz. cream cheese
3/4 tsp. liquid artificial sweetener
1/4 tsp. grated orange rind
1/4 tsp. grated lemon rind
1 tsp. walnuts, chopped
1/4 c. unsweetened moist shredded coconut

Work cream cheese with spoon until light and fluffy. Thoroughly mix in sweetener along with grated fruit rinds and walnuts. Form into 12 balls about 1 inch in diameter. Roll in coconut and refrigerate. Makes 12 cookies.

DATE DROPS

2 eggs, beaten
1/3 c. margarine
1/2 black dates, finely cut
1 1/2 c. crisp rice cereal
1/2 c. nuts, chopped
1 tsp. vanilla

Combine eggs, margarine, and dates. Cook over low heat, stirring constantly. Boil 2 minutes. Remove from heat and add cereal, nuts, and vanilla. Cool. Shape into balls. Makes 42 cookies.

BUTTERSCOTCH SQUARES

1/2 c. diet margarine
Non-nutritive sweetener equivalent to 2 c. brown sugar
1 tsp. vanilla extract
1/2 c. walnuts, chopped
1/2 c. eggs (2 med.)
1 1/2 c. flour
2 tsp. baking powder

Preheat oven to 350 degrees. Cook margarine and sweetener together until smooth. Cool to lukewarm. Add eggs and beat well.

Add flour, baking powder, vanilla, and walnuts. Spread in 9 x 12 x 2 inch pan which has been lightly greased. Bake 1/2 hour. Cut in squares 1 1/4 x 1 1/4 inch. Sprinkle with non-nutritive granulated sugar; cool. Yield: 70 squares.

BROWNIES

1 c. cake flour
1/2 tsp. salt
1 tsp. baking powder
2 tbsp. cocoa
1 oz. melted chocolate
1/2 c. skim milk
1/4 c. vegetable shortening
3 eggs
1/2 c. sugar substitute
1/2 c. nuts, ground or slivered

Sift together first 3 ingredients. Pour melted chocolate over shortening and blend well. Beat eggs until thick and lemon colored. Add sugar substitute; add chocolate mixture and part of dry ingredients. Beat and add remaining dry mixture, alternately with the milk. Fold in nuts. Spread in 2 (8 inch) greased and paper lined pans. Bake at 325 degrees for 17 to 20 minutes. Makes 64 (1 x 2 inch) bars.

DATE COOKIES

1 c. raisins
1/2 c. chopped dates
1 c. water
2 eggs
1/4 c. margarine
1 tbsp. liquid sugar substitute
1 tsp. vanilla
1/4 tsp. cinnamon
1 c. flour
1 tsp. baking soda

Combine in saucepan raisins, dates, and water. Boil 3 minutes; stir constantly. Cool. Cream together eggs, margarine, liquid sugar substitute, and vanilla. Sift together cinnamon, flour, and soda. Add dry ingredients to creamed mixture. Beat well and chill for several hours. Drop from teaspoon onto greased baking sheet. Bake at 350 degrees for 10 to 12 minutes. Yields: 48 (2 inch) cookies.

DIABETIC SPICE COOKIES

1 1/4 c. water
1/3 c. shortening
2 c. raisins or currants
2 tsp. cinnamon
1 tsp. baking powder
1/2 tsp. nutmeg
2 c. flour (approximately)
2 eggs
1/2 tsp. salt
1 tsp. soda
1 tbsp. artificial sweetener

Combine water, shortening, raisins, cinnamon, and nutmeg. Boil for 3 minutes. Cool. Add eggs, one at a time, and beat in salt and soda. Add sweetener, flour, and baking powder. Add flour slowly until mixture is easy to spoon. Blend all ingredients together and drop from teaspoon onto greased cookie sheet. Bake at 350 degrees for 8 to 10 minutes. Makes 4 dozen.

ELEANOR'S THUMBPRINTS

3/4 c. margarine, softened
2 tbsp. sugar
1 1/2 tsp. Sweet 'N Low brown sugar substitute
1 egg
1/2 tsp. vanilla
2 c. all-purpose flour
1/4 tsp. baking powder
1 tbsp. poppy seeds
1/2 c. low sugar strawberry spread

In bowl with mixer, cream margarine, sugar, and Sweet 'N Low. Beat in egg and vanilla. Stir in flour, baking powder, and poppy seeds. Shape dough into ball. Cover; chill about 30 minutes. Preheat oven to 350 degrees. Shape dough into 24 balls. Place 1 inch apart on ungreased baking sheet. Press thumb prints into center of cookies to make deep indentation. Bake about 15 minutes. Fill each cookie with 1 teaspoon strawberry spread. Return to oven and bake 3 minutes. Transfer to wire rack and cool completely. Yield: 24 cookies.

SUGAR FREE OATMEAL COOKIES

3/4 c. vegetable shortening
Sugar Twin equivalent to 1 1/2 c. sugar (or Brown Sugar Twin)
1 egg
1/4 c. water
1 tsp. vanilla
3 c. uncooked oatmeal
1 c. flour
1 tbsp. salt
1/2 tsp. soda

Preheat oven to 350 degrees. Beat together first 5 ingredients. Sift dry ingredients together. Add oatmeal and combine all together. Drop by teaspoon on greased cookie sheet. Bake at 350 degrees for 12 to 15 minutes. Add nuts, raisins, dates, or chocolate chips for variety. Makes 60 cookies.

SESAME LACE COOKIES

5 tbsp. margarine, melted and cooled
Sugar substitute = to 3 tbsp. sugar
2 tbsp. cornstarch
2 tbsp. sesame seeds
1 tbsp. plus 1 1/2 tsp. plain dry bread crumbs
1 tsp. vanilla extract

Preheat oven to 375 degrees. In a bowl, stir all ingredients together until smooth. Drop by teaspoon onto a baking sheet, 4 inches apart. Bake for 7 to 8 minutes until lacy and golden. Let cookies cool on the baking sheet out of the oven for 3 minutes or until easy to lift with a thin metal spatula onto a cooling rack. These are very delicate so handle with care Makes about 2 dz cookies. *Note:* If making cookies small, less baking time is necessary. Check after 5 minutes. *Per serving: 68 calories, 6 gm carbohydrates, trace protein, 5 gm fat, 44 mg sodium. Exchange: 1/2 fruit, 1 fat. Serving size: 2 cookies. Cholesterol: 0 mg per serving.*

PARTY MIX

1/2 c. margarine
1 tsp. garlic powder
2 c. unsalted pretzels
2 c. puffed rice
2 c. spoon-size shredded wheat
2 c. unsalted peanuts

Preheat oven to 250 degrees. Melt margarine in skillet or wok. Add garlic powder,stir then add remaining ingredients and toss together. Serve warm. Makes 2 quarts. Vary the cereals, choosing those which are salt free.

Walnuts and pecans may be used in place of peanuts since a handful of peanuts has 500 calories. 1 cup raisins may also be added but omit garlic powder. Bake party mix a total of 45 minutes. Stir twice during that time period.

DIABETIC ZUCCHINI - BASIL MUFFINS

2 eggs
3/4 c. milk
2/3 c. oil
2 c. flour
Sugar substitute = to 1/4 c. sugar
1 tbsp. baking powder
1 tsp. salt
2 c. shredded zucchini
2 tbsp. minced basil
1/4 c. grated Parmesan cheese

Beat eggs in bowl. Stir in milk and oil. Combine flour, sugar, baking powder and salt. Mix dry ingredients into egg mixture just until flour is moistened. Batter should not be completely smooth. Gently mix in zucchini and basil. Fill greased muffin caps about 3/4 full. Sprinkle with cheese. Bake at 425 degrees for 20-25 minutes. Remove from pan. makes 10-18 muffins depending on size of pan.

DIABETIC CAKE

2 c. water
2 c. raisins
1 c. unsweetened applesauce
2 eggs
2 tbsp. liquid sweetener
3/4 c. oil
1 tsp. baking soda
2 c. flour
1 1/4 tsp. cinnamon
1 tsp. vanilla

Cook raisins in water until all water is absorbed. Mix applesauce, sweetener, eggs, oil together. Then add all other ingredients and stir together. Pour into a greased and floured tube pan. Bake at 350 degrees until tested done with a toothpick.

DIABETIC DATE - NUT CAKE

1 c. butter or margarine
1 tbsp. sucaryl
1 egg
1 c. dates, finely diced
1 1/2 c. or 2 sm. cans diabetic applesauce
1 c. pecans, coarsely chopped
1 tsp. cinnamon
1/2 tsp. cloves
1 tsp. vanilla
2 c. flour
2 tsp. soda

Cream butter, add egg, sucaryl and vanilla which has been beaten together. Sift dry ingredients together and add to other mixture. Beat at medium speed until well blended. Turn into buttered loaf pan and bake at 350 degrees for 1 hour.

DATE COOKIES FOR DIABETICS

1 c. raisins
1/2 c. dates
1 c. water
2 eggs
1/2 c. margarine
3 packets Equal sweetener
1 c. plain flour
1 tsp. soda
1 tsp. cinnamon

Boil raisins, dates and water for 3 minutes; cool. Cream eggs, margarine and Equal. Sift together flour, soda and cinnamon. Combine all ingredients. Beat well and chill several hours or overnight. Drop by teaspoonfuls on a greased cookie sheet. Bake at 350 degrees for 10 minutes.

DIABETIC FRUIT CAKE

1 lb. dates, chopped
1 lb. raisins
2 c. nuts, chopped
1 c. margarine
3 big ripe bananas
1 tsp. nutmeg
6 eggs
3 c. self-rising flour
1 (16 oz.) can crushed pineapple (in own juice) (Separate pineapple&juice, if juice doesn't make1 cup add water)

Mix dates, raisins and nuts with flour, then mix with the rest. Cream bananas, nutmeg and margarine together. Next mix in one egg at a time. Now add 2 cups flour and pineapple juice. Mix well. Put in cold oven at 300 degrees for 2 1/2 hours or less.

DIABETIC COOKIES

2 med. bananas
1/3 c. vegetable oil
1 c. chopped walnuts
2 c. quick oatmeal
1 1/2 tsp. vanilla
1 c. chopped Dates

Mash bananas. Pour oil over top. Mix dates and nuts. Add vanilla and oatmeal. Mix by hand or spoon. Drop onto lightly greased cookie sheet by full teaspoon. Bake at 350 degrees for 25 minutes until lightly browned. Remove at once to rack.

DIABETIC COOKIES

1/2 c. raisins
1/2 c. dates
1 1/2 c. quick oats
1 tsp. cinnamon
1/4 tbsp. soda
1/2 c. flour
1/2 tsp. salt
1 egg
1 tbsp. liquid sweetener (NON - concentrated)
1/4 c. oil
1 tsp. vanilla

Put raisins and dates in small pan and cover with water; bring to boil. Pour off water and set aside. Mix oats, cinnamon, soda, flour and salt in bowl and mix well. Add dry ingredients to date - raisin mixture with egg. Mix and drop onto cookie sheet. Bake at 400 degrees about 8 minutes. Check bottom of cookies during cooking (sometimes the bottom cooks faster than the top).

DIABETIC CAKE

2 c. water
2 c. raisins
1 c. unsweetened applesauce
2 eggs
2 tbsp. artificial sweetener
3/4 c. polyunsaturated cooking oil
1 tsp. baking soda
2 c. flour
1 1/2 tsp. cinnamon
1/2 tsp. nutmeg
1 tsp. vanilla

Cook raisins in 2 cups water until water evaporates. Add applesauce, eggs, sweetener, and cooking oil. Mix well. Blend in baking soda and flour. Add cinnamon, nutmeg and vanilla. Mix well. Pour into greased and floured 8 x 8 inch cake pan. Bake at 350 degrees for 25 minutes or until done.

BEST DIABETIC COOKIE

1/2 c. dates, chopped
1 c. white raisins, chopped
1/2 c. apples, chopped
3/4 c. nuts
1 c. water
1/2 c. margarine
2 eggs, beaten
3 tsp. liquid sweetener
1/2 tsp. vanilla
1 tsp. baking soda
1 c. flour

Boil raisins and apples in the water for 2 or 3 minutes and cool. Then add rest of ingredients; mix. Refrigerate before baking. Bake at 350 degrees.

DIABETIC PEANUT BUTTER COOKIES

2 tsp. liquid sweetener
1 tbsp. butter
1/2 c. peanut butter
2 eggs, slightly beaten
1/2 c. skim milk
1 c. flour
1/4 tsp. baking soda

Melt shortening and peanut butter. Add sweetener and eggs and blend well. Add flour, alternately with milk to which baking soda has been added. Mix well. Drop by teaspoon on ungreased cookie sheet. Bake at 375 degrees for 15 minutes. Amount -40. Exchange -2 cookies = 1 milk. Calories -2 cookies = 75.

DIABETIC COOKIES

2 tsp. cinnamon
1 tsp. soda
2 eggs
1/2 c. oil
1 c. rolled oats
1 c. raisins
1 tsp. nutmeg
1/2 tsp. Cloves
1/2 tsp. salt
1 c. unsweetened applesauce
1 tsp. liquid sweetener
1 sm. can pineapple, crushed (natural & drained)

Preheat oven to 350 degrees Mix dry ingredients then add remaining ingredients. Drop by teaspoon or tablespoon onto greased cookie sheets. Bake for approx. 5-10 min. They bake fast so test by pressing (ovens temps may vary). Should be refrigerated (they grow mold easily so store in air-tight container). *2 or 3 small cookies = 1 bread exchange. 1 or 2 larger cookies = 1 bread exchange*

DIABETIC RAISIN COOKIES

1/4 c. non-fat dry milk
1/4 c. ice water
1/2 c. raisins
1/2 c. margarine
1/2 c. brown sugar twin
1 egg
1 tsp. vanilla
1 c. flour
1 tsp. cinnamon
1/2 tsp. baking soda
1/2 tsp. salt
1 c. rolled oats

Whip non-fat dry milk with ice water until stiff peaks form (4 to 5 minutes). Boil raisins in water for 2 minutes, drain. Combine margarine, sugar twin, egg and vanilla. Beat 1 minute at medium speed. Stir into dry ingredients raisin liquid. Beat 2 minutes. Stir in rolled oats and raisins. Fold in whipped non-fat milk. Drop from teaspoon 2 inches apart onto non-greased cookie sheet. Bake at 375 degrees for 15 to 20 minutes.

DIABETIC COOKIES

1 3/4 c. flour
1 tsp. cinnamon
1/2 tsp. nutmeg
1/2 tsp. cloves
1 tsp. baking soda
1/2 c. (1 stick) margarine
1/2 c. Sugar Twin
1 egg
1 c. applesauce, unsweetened
1/2 c. raisins, chopped
1 c. All Bran Buds
1/2 c. finely chopped nuts

Preheat oven to 350 degrees. Sift together flour, cinnamon, nutmeg, cloves, and baking soda. In large bowl, mix together margarine, artificial sweetener, and egg. Mix in dry ingredients, alternating with applesauce. Fold in bran, raisins, and nuts; mix thoroughly. Drop onto greased cookie sheet by tablespoon. Lightly flatten with fork, dipped in milk. Bake for 7 to 8 minutes. *Makes 36 cookies. Exchanges: 1 cookie = 1 fat and 1/2 bread exchange. Calories: 76 calories per cookie.*

DIABETIC DATE NUT CAKE

1/2 c. butter or oleo, softened
1 tbsp. liquid sweetener
1 egg
1 c. chopped nuts
1 c. chopped dates
1 1/2 c. diet applesauce
1/2 tsp. cinnamon
1/4 tsp. cloves
1 tsp. vanilla
1 tsp. soda
2 c. flour

Cream butter or oleo. Add egg, sweetener and vanilla; mix well. Sift dry ingredients together and add to other mixture. Stir in dates, applesauce and pecans. After everything has been mixed, beat with a mixer at medium speed or until well blended. Turn into a greased and floured loaf pan and bake at 350 degrees for nearly an hour.

DIABETIC COOKIES

3/4 c. shortening
4 tsp. liquid sweetener
1 c. sifted flour
1/2 tsp. nutmeg
1 tsp. vanilla
2 sm. bananas, mashed
1 tsp. soda
1 egg, well beaten
1/2 c. boiling water
1/4 tsp. salt
1/2 c. finely chopped nuts
3/4 c. quick oats

1/2 c. dates or raisins

Pour boiling water over dates or raisins. Let set while mixing other ingredients. Add fruit and mix well. Drop by teaspoon on greased cookie sheet. Bake about 12 minutes at 375 degrees.

APPLESAUCE DIABETIC CAKE

2 sticks oleo
2 tbsp. sweetener
1 1/2 c. applesauce (unsweetened)
1 egg
1 c. raisins
2 c. flour
2 tsp. soda
1 tsp. vanilla

Bake in loaf pan at 350 - 375 degrees for 45 to 60 minutes.

LOW SUGAR DIABETIC CAKE

2 c. golden raisins
2 eggs, beaten
2 tbsp. liquid sweetener, Sweet 10
1 tsp. soda
1 tsp. vanilla
1/2 tsp. nutmeg
1 c. unsweetened applesauce
2 c. water
3/4 c. vegetable oil
1 1/4 tsp. cinnamon
2 c. all-purpose flour

Boil raisins in water until all water is absorbed and then cool. Add applesauce, eggs, liquid sweetener and vegetable oil. Mix well. Blend in soda, flour, cinnamon, nutmeg and vanilla. Mix well. Pour into greased tube pan and bake at 350 degrees for 50 to 60 minutes or until test done. Serves 20. Each serving equals 1 bread, 1/2 fruit and 1 1/2 fat exchange.

DIABETIC POUND CAKE

2 c. flour
1/2 c. corn oil
2 eggs
3 lg. ripe bananas
1 tsp. vanilla
1 tsp. soda
1 1/2 tbsp. liquid sugar substitute
4 tbsp. buttermilk
1 c. raisins
1 1/2 c. pecans

Sift flour and soda. Add oil, sugar substitute and mix well until light. Beat eggs and add rest of ingredients. Beat until well mixed. Pour into loaf pan and bake at 350 degrees for 25 minutes.

DIABETIC PUMPKIN COOKIES

1 c. shortening
1 egg
2 c. flour
1/2 tsp. nutmeg
1 tsp. baking powder
1 c. cooked pumpkin
1 tsp. vanilla
1/4 tsp. allspice
1/2 tsp. baking soda
1 tsp. cinnamon
1 c. raisins
1/2 c. nuts, chopped

Soak raisins in hot water for 5 minutes. Drain. Cream shortening. Add pumpkin, egg and vanilla. Beat well. Mix dry ingredients. Add to creamed mixture. Mix well. Add raisins and nuts. Drop onto greased cookie sheets and press with a fork. Bake at 350 degrees for 12 minutes. Freeze them as otherwise they will get moldy. Yields 3 to 4 dozen cookies.

DIABETIC DATE NUT CAKE

1 c. butter or margarine
1 egg
1 tbsp. liquid sweetener
2 tsp. soda
1/4 tsp. cloves
1/2 tsp. cinnamon
1 c. dates, cut fine
1 1/2 c. applesauce
1 c. pecans, broken
1 tsp. vanilla
2 c. flour

Cream butter , add egg, sweetener and vanilla. Sift together all dry ingredients. Add applesauce, dates and pecans.

DIABETIC FROSTING

1/4 c. cream cheese
2 tsp. skim milk
Sweetener equivalent to 1/4 c. powdered sugar
1/4 tsp. salt
1/2 tsp. vanilla
Food coloring

Cream cheese and milk thoroughly. Add sweetener, salt and vanilla. Add coloring last, if desired. Makes 1/3 cup frosting.

DIABETIC DATE COFFEE CAKE

1/3 c. mashed bananas
1/2 c. butter
3 lg. eggs
1 tsp. vanilla extract
1 1/4 c. water
3 c. unbleached flour
1 tsp. baking soda

2 tsp. baking powder
1 1/2 c. chopped dates

--TOPPING--
1/3 c. chopped dates
1/3 c. chopped walnuts
1/3 c. flaked coconut

Beat together mashed bananas and butter until creamy. Add eggs, vanilla, and water. Beat and measure flour, baking soda, and baking powder. Stir in 1 1/2 cup of dates. Spoon batter into an oiled and floured 9x13 inch baking pan and spread evenly. Combine topping and sprinkle over batter. Bake at 350 degrees for 20-25 minutes or until a knife comes out clean. Cool on wire rack.

DIABETIC APPLESAUCE CAKE

1 stick margarine, melted & cooled
1 1/2 c. unsweetened applesauce
1 egg, beaten
2 c. self-rising flour
1 tsp. soda
1/2 tsp. cinnamon
1/4 tsp. cloves
1/2 tsp. salt
2 tsp. sugar twin
3 tsp. lemon flavor
1 1/2 c. raisins, chopped & floured
1/2 c. chopped nuts

Blend together margarine, applesauce and egg. Sift together flour, soda, spices and salt. Add sugar twin; add to mixture and heat well. Stir in lemon flavor. Fold in raisins and nuts. Pour into well greased and floured tube pan. Bake in preheated 350 degree oven for 30 minutes. Do not overbake.

DIABETIC COOKIES

1 stick margarine
1/4 c. milk
1 block unsweetened chocolate
1 box ground dates (optional)
1 box chopped raisins
1 c. chopped nuts
1/2 c. peanut butter
1 tsp. liquid sweetener
3 c. quick cooking oatmeal
1 tsp. vanilla

Cook margarine, milk and chocolate for 1 minute. Stir while cooking. Add raisins, nuts, peanut butter, sweetener, oatmeal and vanilla. Mix together with hands. Roll into walnut size balls. Makes 40 cookies at 120 calories each. Do not bake. May be frozen.

DIABETIC DIET COOKIES

1 2/3 c. plain flour
1 tsp. soda
1/2 tsp. salt or salt substitute
2 tsp. apple pie spice
1 c. diet margarine
6 tbsp. or 6 packs sugar substituted (such as Sweet 'N Low)
1 tsp. vanilla
1 egg
1 c. unsweetened applesauce
2/3 c. raisins
1 c. All Bran cereal

Sift flour, salt, soda, and spices. Beat margarine, sugar substitute, vanilla, and egg until blended. Mixture will be rough and crumbly due to the margarine. Add dry ingredients and applesauce. Mix well after each addition. Stir in cereal and raisins. Bake in 9 x 13 inch pan at 375 degrees for about 15 minutes. Cool and cut in blocks. Can be frozen. About 23 calories per cookies.

DIABETIC CAKE

1/2 c. margarine
1 egg
1 tbsp. liquid artificial sweetener
1 tsp. vanilla
2 c. flour
2 tsp. soda
1/2 tsp. cinnamon
1/4 tsp. ground cloves
1 c. chopped dates
1 3/4 c. unsweetened applesauce
1 c. chopped nuts

Cream margarine; add egg, sweetener and vanilla. Sift together dry ingredients and add to mixture. Add applesauce, dates and nuts. Beat with electric mixer on high speed for several minutes until well blended. Bake in Bundt pan at 325 degrees for 1 hour or until done.

DIABETIC CAKE

2 c. water
2 c. raisins
1 c. unsweetened applesauce
2 c. flour
1 tsp. vanilla
2 eggs
2 tbsp. liquid sweetener
3/4 c. cooking oil
1 tsp. baking soda
1 1/4 tsp. cinnamon
1/2 tsp. nutmeg

Cook raisins in water until water is gone. Cool. Then add applesauce, eggs, sweetener and oil. Mix well. Blend in baking soda and flour. Add remaining ingredients and mix well. You may add walnuts, or artificially sweetened fruit cocktail may be used instead of raisins, if desired. Bake at 350 degrees for about 40 minutes or more.

DIABETIC COOKIES

1 1/4 c. water
1 tsp. nutmeg
2 tsp. cinnamon
1/2 tsp. salt
2 c. raisins
1/2 c. shortening

Boil all ingredients for 3 minutes and let cool. Add:
2 eggs
2 tbsp. water
2 c. sifted flour
1/4 c. brown sugar substitute
1/4 c. white sugar substitute
1 tsp. baking powder
1 tsp. baking soda

Drop by teaspoonful on greased cookie sheet. Bake for 10-12 minutes at 350 degrees.

BROWNIES FOR DIABETICS

1/2 c. margarine
3 scant tsp. liquid sweetener
2 sq. unsweetened melted chocolate
3/4 c. sifted flour
1/2 c. chopped walnuts
2 eggs
1 tsp. vanilla
1 tsp. baking powder

Cream margarine, sweetener, and chocolate, beat until smooth. Beat in eggs and vanilla; add flour, baking powder, and walnuts. Beat until smooth. Spread batter in greased 8 x 8 inch pan and bake at 350 degrees for 30 minutes. Cool in pan.

DIABETIC COOKIES

1 1/4 c. water
1 1/4 c. shortening
2 c. seedless raisins
1/2 tsp. nutmeg
2 tsp. cinnamon

Boil all of the above for 3 minutes. Let cool. Beat in 2 eggs. Dissolve 1/2 teaspoon salt, 1 teaspoon soda, 12 1/4 ground saccarin in 2 tablespoons water. Add to above mix and add 2 cups flour and 1 teaspoon baking powder. Bake at 350 degrees for 10-12 minutes.

DIABETIC APPLE CAKE

2/3 c. oil
5 tbsp. sugar substitute
1 egg
1 tsp. vanilla
1/2 tsp. salt
1 tsp. baking powder
1/2 tsp. baking soda
1 1/2 c. flour
1/2 c. raisins
1/2 c. water
1 1/2 c. chopped apples

Mix all ingredients. Pour into a lightly greased 9 x 9 inch pan. Sprinkle with nuts. Bake at 350 degrees for 30 minutes. Makes 16 servings. You can substitute carrots, bananas and pumpkin for the apples. All works well, can also be made into cupcakes.

DIABETIC CAKE

2 c. Bisquick
1 c. dates (cut up)
1 c. raisins
1 c. prunes (steamed and chopped)
1 c. applesauce
1/2 c. walnuts

2 tbsp. soft butter
1/2 tsp. soda
2 eggs

Combine all ingredients, putting the soda in the applesauce. Bake about 30 minutes at 300 degrees.

DIABETIC APPLESAUCE CAKE

1 stick margarine, melted
1 1/2 c. unsweetened applesauce
1 egg, beaten
2 c. flour
1 tsp. soda
1/2 tsp. cinnamon
1/4 tsp. cloves
Dash of nutmeg
1-2 tsp. Sugar Twin
1 1/2 c. chopped dates
1/2 c. pecans
1 c. raisins

Blend together margarine, applesauce and egg. Sift flour and all dry ingredients together. Add them to mixture, stir in vanilla and fold in dates and nuts. Bake in a well greased floured tube pan in preheated oven at 350 degrees for 30 minutes. Do not over bake.

BANANA RAISIN CAKE FOR DIABETICS

2 c. flour
1 1/2 tsp. baking powder
Non Nutrive sweetener equivalent to 11/2 c. sugar, 6 tsp. Sweet & low
1 tsp. soda
1 tsp. salt
1/2 c. diet margarine
1 c. banana, about 3 mashed
1 tsp. lemon peel grated
1 tsp. vanilla extract
2 eggs
1 c. white raisins, chopped

1/2 c. nuts, chopped fine

Preheat oven to 350 degrees and bake 1 hour 20 minutes or until done.

DIABETIC CAKE

2 c. water
2 c. raisins
1 c. unsweetened applesauce
3/4 c. polyunsaturated oil
1 tsp. baking soda
1 c. flour*
1 c. oats*
1 1/2 tsp. cinnamon
1/2 tsp. nutmeg
2 eggs
2 tbsp. artificial sweetened
1 tsp. vanilla
1/2 c. pecans

*Or use 2 cups flour and no oats. Cook raisins in 2 cups of water until water evaporates. Add applesauce, eggs, sweetener and oil. Mix well, mix together flour, baking soda and spices. Blend into raisins, add vanilla and mix well. Pour into a greased and floured 8x8 inch cake pan. Bake at 350 degrees for 25 or 30 minutes. Refrigerate after first day. Cake without sugar spoils easily.

OATMEAL RAISIN COOKIES - DIABETIC

1/2 c. margarine
1 egg
3/4 c. flour
1 c. oatmeal
1/4 tsp. salt
1/2 tsp. soda
1 1/4 tsp. liquid artificial sweetener
1 tsp. vanilla

1/4 c. raisins
5 tbsp. orange juice concentrate, undiluted

Mix all ingredients together and drop by teaspoonfuls onto cookie sheet, flatten. Bake at 350 degrees for 15-20 minutes. Yields: about 40 cookies. Exchange: 2 cookies = 1/2 bread.

DIABETIC CAKE

1/2 stick oleo
2 eggs
1 tbsp. Sucryl
1 tsp. vanilla
1 1/2 c. unsweetened applesauce
1/4 tsp. cinnamon
1/4 tsp. cloves
2 tsp. soda
1 c. pecans
1 c. chopped dates
2 c. flour

DIABETIC COOKIES

1 c. water
1/3 c. oil
2 c. seedless raisins
2 c. flour
2 tsp. cinnamon
1/2 tsp. nutmeg
2 eggs
1 tsp. baking powder
1 tsp. salt
1 tsp. soda
1/2 c. chopped nuts
2 tbsp. sweetener and water

Put water, oil, raisins and spices in saucepan and boil for 3 minutes. When cool, add remaining ingredients and drop by teaspoons on cookie sheet. Bake at 350 degrees until done.

DIABETIC POUND CAKE

2 c. flour
1/2 c. corn oil
2 eggs
3 lg. ripe bananas
1 1/2 tbsp. liquid sweetener
4 tbsp. buttermilk
1 c. raisins
1 tsp. soda
1 tsp. vanilla
1 1/2 c. pecans

Sift flour and soda. Add oil, liquid sweetener. Mix well until light. Beat in eggs. Add rest of ingredients. Beat until well mixed. Pour into loaf pan. Bake at 350 degrees for 25 minutes.

DIABETIC COOKIES

1 1/2 c. unsweetened applesauce
3/4 c. margarine
2 eggs
2 tbsp. cinnamon
1/2 tsp. allspice
1 1/2 c. flour
1 1/2 tsp. soda
1 tbsp. vanilla
1/3 c. brown Sugar Twin
2 c. oatmeal
1/2 tsp. salt
1 c. raisins
1/4 c. nuts

Mix applesauce, margarine, eggs, vanilla and Sugar Twin. Add the remaining ingredients. Drop by teaspoonfuls onto cookie sheet and bake 15 minutes at 375 degrees.

DIABETIC MOLASSES COOKIES

1/2 c. vegetable oil
1/4 c. molasses
1/4 c. sugar
1 egg
2 c. whole wheat flour
2 tsp. baking soda
1 tsp. ground cinnamon
1/2 tsp. ground ginger
1/4 tsp. cloves

Beat together the oil, the molasses, sugar and egg. Add the remaining ingredients and mix well. Chill dough for 2 hours or overnight.

DIABETIC ORANGE RAISIN CLUSTERS

1/3 c. vegetable oil
1/4 c. sugar
1 egg
2 c. whole wheat flour
2 1/2 tsp. baking powder
1 1/2 tsp. ground cinnamon
1/2 tsp. baking soda
1/4 tsp. ground cloves
1/3 c. frozen undiluted orange juice concentrate
1/4 c. honey
1 c. raisins
1 c. uncooked oats
1/4 c. sunflower seeds

Combine oil and sugar. Beat well. Add egg. Stir in flour, baking powder, cinnamon, baking soda, cloves, orange juice concentrate and honey.

DIABETIC COOKIES

1 3/4 c. flour
1 tsp. cinnamon
1/2 tsp. cloves
1/2 tsp. nutmeg
1 tsp. baking soda
1/2 c. (1 stick) margarine
1/2 c. Sugar Twin
1 egg
1 c. applesauce (unsweetened)
1/2 c. raisins (chopped)
1 c. All-Bran Buds
1/2 c. finely chopped nuts

Preheat oven to 350 degrees. Sift together flour, cinnamon, nutmeg, cloves and baking soda. In large bowl, mix together margarine, artificial sweetener and egg. Mix in dry ingredients, alternating with applesauce. Fold in bran, raisins and nuts and mix thoroughly.

PEANUT BUTTER COOKIES

1 c. flour
1/2 c. creamy peanut butter
1 egg
1 tsp. vanilla
1/4 tsp. salt
1 1/2 tsp. baking powder
1/2 c. water
1 tbsp. liquid sweetener
1/2 c. salad oil

Mix all together in a large bowl. Shape into balls and place on an ungreased cookie sheet. Bake at 375 degrees for 12 to 15 minutes. You may add a little more flour if desired.

DIABETIC OATMEAL FRUIT DROP COOKIES

1/2 c. butter or oleo
1 tbsp. vanilla
1/4 c. white flour
1/2 tbsp. salt
1/2 c. dried fruit (figs, dates,
   raisins, cut small)
1 c. quick uncooked oatmeal
2 eggs
1/4 c. whole wheat flour
1/2 tbsp. baking powder
Granular sweetener to equal
1/2 c. sugar
1/2 c. chopped walnuts

Melt butter, beat in eggs and vanilla. Sift together flours and baking powder. Add salt, sugar, fruit, nuts and oatmeal. Stir until blended. Drop by teaspoon onto greased cookie sheet. Bake at 350 degrees for 12 to 15 minutes.

DIABETIC RAISIN DROP COOKIES

1 1/4 c. hot water
1/2 tsp. nutmeg
1 tbsp. water
1 tsp. baking powder
1/2 c. oleo
2 tsp. cinnamon
1 tsp. Sweetener
1/2 tsp. salt
2 c. raisins
2 eggs, beaten
2 c. flour

Heat oven to 350 degrees. Grease cookie sheets. Combine hot water, oleo, raisins and let cool. Mix other ingredients together and add to first mixture. Drop by teaspoonsful on greased cookie sheet floured and bake for 15 to 18 minutes.

DIABETIC LEMON COCONUT COOKIES

1 stick oleo
1 egg
1/2 tsp. salt
2 tbsp. sweetener
2 tbsp. bottled lemon juice
1 c. coconut
1 1/2 c. flour
1/2 tsp. soda
1 tsp. baking powder

Mix oleo, egg and next 5 ingredients. Mix well. Add flour and coconut.
Mix thoroughly and drop by spoonfuls onto greased cookie sheet.
Bake at 350 degrees for 18 to 19 minutes. 3 cookies = 1 bread
exchange.

DIABETIC COOKIES

1 1/2 c. butter or oleo
2/3 c. Sprinkle Sweet
3/4 c. buttermilk
2 eggs
1 tsp. soda
1 tsp. baking powder
2 c. flour
1 c. raisins
1 c. dates
1 c. nut meats (optional)

Follow directions as listed only put 1 teaspoon soda with the sour milk.
Bake at 375 degrees for 10 minutes.

OATMEAL APPLESAUCE MUFFINS - DIABETIC

1/2 c. unsweetened applesauce
1/2 c. skim milk
3/4 c. dry quick cook oatmeal
2 tbsp. oil
3/4 c. flour
2 lg. eggs
2 tsp. vanilla
2 tsp. cinnamon
1 tsp. ginger
2 tsp. baking powder
1/2 tsp. salt
5 tsp. brown sugar

Combine oatmeal, applesauce, milk and oil. Let stand for 20 minutes. In another bowl combine flour, cinnamon, ginger, salt and baking powder. Add slightly beaten eggs, vanilla and brown sugar to oatmeal mixture. Add dry ingredients. Stir just enough to moisten. Spray muffin tins with vegetables spray. Fill tins 2/3 full. Bake at 350 degrees for 15-20 minutes.

DIABETIC NUT CAKE

1/2 c. oleo
1 egg
1 tbsp. liquid sweetener
1 tsp. vanilla
2 c. flour
2 tsp. soda
1/2 tsp. cloves
1/2 tsp. cinnamon
1 c. dates, cut fine
1 1/2 c. unsweetened applesauce
1 c. pecans

Cream oleo. Add egg, sweetener and vanilla; mix. Sift flour, soda, cloves and cinnamon. Add to first mixture. Stir applesauce, dates and pecans in last. Bake in pans or loaf for 1 hour at 350 degrees.

DIABETIC GRANOLA BARS

1 env. chocolate Alba 77 shake mix
3 tbsp. water
1/4 c. Grape Nut flakes
2 tbsp. chunky peanut butter
2 tbsp. raisins

Mix Alba 77 with water. Add remaining ingredients. Form 2x5 inch bars on aluminum foil and freeze for 2 hours.

DIABETIC CAKE

1 c. raisins
1 c. prunes
1 c. unsweetened applesauce
2 eggs
3/4 c. oil
1/4 c. Sweet and Low (42 pks.)
2 c. self rising flour
1 tsp. cinnamon
1 tsp. soda
1 tsp. nutmeg
1 c. walnuts
1 tsp. vanilla

Cook raisins and prunes in 1 cup of water. Let cool. Beat eggs and applesauce. Combine all other ingredients and bake at 350 degrees for 30-40 minutes in sheet pan.

DIABETIC CAKE

2 c. water
2 c. raisins
1 can unsweetened applesauce
3/4 c. cooking oil
1/2 tsp. vanilla

1 c. chopped nuts
1/2 tsp. nutmeg
1 1/4 tsp. cinnamon
2 tbsp. liquid sweetener
2 eggs
2 c. flour
1 tsp. baking soda

Cook raisins in water until water is gone. Add applesauce, eggs, sweetener, and oil; mix well. Blend in soda and flour. Add remaining ingredients and mix well. Bake at 350 degrees for 35 minutes.

DIABETIC COOKIES

3 med. bananas, mashed
1 tsp. vanilla
1 1/4 c. chopped walnuts
1/3 c. oil
2 c. rolled oats
1/4 c. raisins

Combine bananas, oil, and vanilla. Stir in oats, walnuts, and raisins. Drop by tablespoonfuls onto greased cookie sheet. Press lightly with fork. Bake 10-12 minutes until golden brown at 350 degrees.

DIABETIC FRUIT BARS

1 c. chopped dates
1/2 c. chopped prunes
1/2 c. raisins
1 c. water

Boil 5 minutes and add 1 stick oleo. Let cool. Add: 1 tsp. vanilla 1 c. flour 1 tsp. soda 1/2 c. nuts   Bake for 25 minutes at 350 degrees in a 9x13 Pyrex dish.

DIABETIC UNBAKED FRUIT CAKE

1 box graham cracker crumbs
1 box (8 oz.) dates
1 sm. jar maraschino cherries
1/2 c. golden raisins
1/2 c. raisins
2 pkg. diced dried fruit mix
1 c. pecans
2 (8 oz.) cans crushed pineapple in own juice

Drain cherries and discard liquid. Place in small saucepan. Add enough water to cover. Let come to a boil; drain and repeat. Drain again and cover with cold water. Drain and chop dates, pecans, add diced fruit then add graham cracker crumbs. Drain juice from pineapple reserving juice from 1 can. Pour juice and pineapple over fruit and cracker crumbs. Mix thoroughly until all is moistened. Empty mixture in loaf pan sprayed with non-stick spray, cover with wax paper and press firmly in pan. Chill several hours or freeze before cutting. Yield 40 servings. Exchanges: 1 fruit, 1/2 bread, 1/2 fat, calories 111, carb. 21, protein 1.5 gm., Sodium 56 mg., fat 3 gm.

DIABETIC PUMPKIN BARS

1 1/4 c. flour
1/2 c. margarine
3/4 c. Sugar Twin
3 eggs
1 1/4 tsp. baking powder
1 (16 oz.) can pumpkin
2 tsp. cinnamon
1/2 c. raisins

Cream flour, shortening and Sugar Twin together. Add eggs, pumpkin, and baking powder. Stir until smooth. Add raisins. Bake at 350 degrees for 45 minutes. Sprinkle top with chopped nuts, if desired.

DIABETIC EASTER FUDGE

1 sq. unsweetened chocolate
1/4 c. evaporated milk
1/2 tsp. vanilla
1 tsp. artificial liquid sweetener
1 pkg. vanilla or chocolate artificially sweetened pudding powder (or 8 tsp. finely chopped nuts)

Melt chocolate in top of double boiler over boiling water. Add evaporated milk and mix. Cook 2-3 minutes, then add vanilla and sweetener. Spread on small foil pie pan or plate. Chill. Cut into 8 pieces. Form into egg shaped balls and then roll lightly in pudding powder or chopped nuts.

DIABETIC COOKIES

1 1/2 c. unsweetened applesauce
3/4 c. margarine
2 eggs
1 tbsp. vanilla
1/3 c. Brown Sugar Twin
2 c. oatmeal
1 tbsp. cinnamon
1/2 tsp. allspice
1 1/2 c. flour
1 1/2 tsp. soda
1/2 tsp. salt
1 c. raisins
1/4 c. nuts

Mix the first 5 ingredients well; add the remaining ingredients. Drop by teaspoonfuls onto cookie sheet and bake 15 minutes at 375 degrees.

DIABETIC NUT COOKIES

1/2 c. flour
1/4 tsp. baking powder
1/8 tsp. salt
1/2 tsp. Sweet 'N Low
2 tbsp. unsweetened orange juice
1/2 tsp. vanilla
2 tbsp. vegetable shortening
2 tbsp. chopped nut meats
2 tbsp. grated orange rind

Mix together first 7 ingredients and stir well. Add nut meats and orange rind. Drop by large teaspoonfuls on greased cookie sheet. Bake at 350 degrees for 10 minutes.

DIABETIC CAKE

2 c. raisins
1 1/2 c. water
1/2 c. orange juice
1 c. unsweetened applesauce
2 eggs, beaten (or Eggbeaters)
2 tbsp. liquid sweetener
1/2 c. cooking oil
2 c. self-rising flour
1 tsp. baking soda
1 tsp. cinnamon
1/2 tsp. nutmeg
1 tsp. vanilla

Slowly boil raisins in water until water is absorbed. Add orange juice, applesauce, sweetener, eggs and oil; mix well. Blend flour, baking soda, cinnamon and nutmeg; add to first mixture together with vanilla. Mix well. Pour into greased 9-inch pan. Bake at 350 degrees for 25-30 minutes.

OATMEAL & APPLESAUCE DIABETIC COOKIES

1/2 c. flour
1 1/2 tsp. cinnamon
1/2 tsp. soda
1/4 tsp. salt
1/4 tsp. nutmeg
1 tsp. allspice
1/2 c. oatmeal
1/2 c. raisins
1/2 c. unsweetened applesauce
1/4 c. cooking oil
1 egg
1 tsp. vanilla

Mix flour, cinnamon, soda, salt, nutmeg, allspice, oatmeal and raisins. Add applesauce, egg, oil and vanilla. Mix to moisten and drop onto greased cookie sheet. Bake 12 minutes at 375 degrees.

DIABETIC DATE CAKE

1/2 c. butter
1 tbsp. liquid sweetener or 1/2 c. sugar
1 egg
1 c. finely sliced dates or raisins
1 1/2 c. diabetic applesauce
1 c. chopped pecans (optional)
1/4 tsp. cloves
1 tsp. vanilla
2 c. flour
2 tsp. soda
1/2 tsp. cinnamon

Cream butter, egg and applesauce. Add liquid sweetener and vanilla. Sift dry ingredients together; add to creamed mixture. Beat until well blended. Turn into loaf pan and bake at 350 degrees for 1 hour.

DIABETIC DATE BARS

1 c. chopped dates
1/3 c. vegetable oil
1/2 c. orange juice
1/4 tsp. artificial sweetener
1 c. flour
1 tsp. baking powder
1/2 c. chopped pecans
1/4 c. Eggbeaters (or 1 egg)
1 tbsp. grated orange rind

Boil dates, oil, and orange juice for 5 minutes and cool; add rest of ingredients. Mix all together and spread in oiled 8 x 8 inch baking dish. Bake at 350 degrees for 25 minutes. Cool before cutting. Yields 36 bars. Each bar: 56 calories. 7 grams carbohydrates, 1 gram protein, 3 grams fat, 8 mg. cholesterol, 12 mg. sodium.

DIABETIC COOKIES

1 c. all-purpose flour
1 c. quick oats
3/4 c. seedless raisins
1/2 c. orange juice
1/2 c. butter or margarine, softened
2 tsp. baking powder
1 tsp. grated orange peel
1/2 tsp. salt
1/2 tsp. cinnamon
1 egg
3/4 c. nuts
Sugar substitute to taste

Mix all dry ingredients plus oats, raisins and orange peel. Add orange juice, egg, oil and vanilla. Then add nuts. Mix to moisten and drop onto greased cookie sheet. Bake 12 minutes at 375 degrees.

DIABETIC FRUIT BARS

1 1/4 c. flour
1 c. quick oats
1/2 tsp. salt
1 tbsp. liquid food sweetener
1 tsp. vanilla
1/2 c. vegetable shortening
2 c. drained unsweetened canned fruit such as apples, cherries
3 tbsp. fruit juice

Mix flour, oats, salt, sweetener, vanilla and vegetable shortening with fork until crumbly. Add juices to let crumbs stick together. Spread half on bottom of square pan. Place layer of fruit, spread rest of crumbs on top. Bake, cool and cut in squares.

DIABETIC APPLESAUCE CAKE

1/2 c. water
1/2 c. raisins
1 c. unsweetened applesauce
2 eggs
2 tbsp. liquid sweetener or powder to equal 1 c.
1/2 c. oil
2 c. flour
1 tsp. soda
2 tsp. cinnamon
1/2 tsp. nutmeg
1 tsp. vanilla

Preheat oven to 350 degrees. Cook raisins in water until water evaporates. Add applesauce, eggs, sweetener and oil; mix well. Blend in soda and flour. Add nutmeg, cinnamon and vanilla. Bake in greased loaf pan 4 x 8 x 4 inches for 50 minutes at 350 degrees. Artificially sweetened fruit cocktail may be substituted for raisins to be more like fruitcake.

CHOCOLATE CAKE FOR THE DIABETIC

1 1/2 c. flour
1 1/2 tsp. soda
1/3 c. Sugar Twin + 1 tbsp.
7 pkgs. Equal
1/3 c. cocoa
1 tsp. salt (or less)
1 tbsp. vinegar
1/3 c. oil
1 c. water
1 tsp. oil
1/4 c. buttermilk
2 beaten eggs

Sift dry ingredients together in bowl. Beat eggs and add to rest of ingredients. Stir with fork (don't beat). Pour into loaf pan and bake at 350 degrees for 35 to 40 minutes (test with toothpick).

FRUIT COOKIES FOR DIABETICS

1 c. water
1/3 c. oil
2 c. seedless raisins
2 tbsp. cinnamon
1/2 tsp. nutmeg
1/2 tsp. salt
2 c. flour
1 tsp. baking soda
2 tsp. liquid sweetener
2 tbsp. water
2 beaten eggs
1 tsp. baking powder
1/3 c. chopped nuts

Combine water, oil, raisins, cinnamon, and nutmeg; boil together for 3 minutes. Let cool. Dissolve salt and soda in combined liquid sweetener and water; add to beaten eggs. Stir into cooled mixture. Add flour and baking powder which have been sifted together; mix well. Add nuts, then mix. Drop by teaspoonfuls onto greased cookie sheet. Bake at 375 degrees until lightly browned. Makes 3 dozen cookies.

DIABETIC CAKE

3 lg. eggs
1/2 c. soft butter
1 c. unsweetened pineapple juice
2 1/2 c. unbleached white flour
3 c. grated carrots
1 tsp. soda
2 tsp. baking powder
1 tsp. nutmeg
1 tsp. cinnamon

--TOPPING--
1 c. crushed, drained pineapple
1 tsp. cinnamon

Beat together eggs, butter and pineapple juice. Add flour, soda,
baking powder and spices. Beat well. Stir in grated carrots and mix
well. Pour mixture into greased and floured 9x13 inch pan. Mix
drained pineapple and cinnamon and sprinkle over cake mixture. Bake
25-30 minutes at 350 degrees or until brown.

DIABETIC BLUEBERRY JAM

2 tbsp. lemon juice
3 tsp. unflavored gelatin
1/8 tsp. salt
1 1/2 tsp. arrowroot
2 1/2 c. frozen unsweetened blueberries, partially thawed
Non-nutritive sweetener equivalent to 2 c. sugar

Mix lemon juice, gelatin, salt and arrowroot; stir in blueberries. Boil
gently until mixture thickens, stirring constantly (about 3-4 minutes).
Stir constantly, boiling at full boil for 2 minutes. Remove from heat;
stir in sweetener. Fill and seal jars.

DIABETIC STRAWBERRY JAM

1 c. sliced strawberries
3/4 c. sugar free strawberry soda
1 pkg. strawberry low-calorie Jello
3 packets sugar substitute

Mash strawberries; add soda and bring to a boil, cook 1 minute. Remove from heat; stir in Jello until dissolved. Stir in sugar. Pour into hot jars, seal or store in refrigerator. Exchanges per 1 tablespoon: free. Makes 1 1/2 cups.

DIABETIC CRANBERRY-ORANGE RELISH

2 c. cranberries
Sweet 'n Low to equal 1 c. sugar
1 orange

Grind fruit, blend in sweetener; chill well. 8 servings, 24 calories each. 1 serving = 1/2 fruit exchange.

DIABETIC'S PUMPKIN PIE

1 baked & cooled 9" pie shell
2 sm. pkg. sugar-free instant vanilla pudding
2 c. milk
1 c. canned pumpkin
1 tsp. pumpkin pie spice
1/4 tsp. nutmeg
1/4 tsp. ginger
1/2 tsp. cinnamon

Blend all ingredients in blender until smooth. Use plain canned pumpkin. Do not use canned pumpkin pie mixture. Pour into pie shell and chill until ready to serve.

DIABETIC RAISIN APPLESAUCE CAKE

2 c. water
2 c. raisins
1 c. unsweetened applesauce
1 1/2 tsp. diabetic brown sweetener
3/4 c. cooking oil
1 tsp. baking soda
2 c. flour
1 1/4 tsp. cinnamon
2 eggs
1/2 tsp. nutmeg
1 tsp. vanilla
1/2 tsp. salt

Cook raisins in water until the water is gone. Cool. Add applesauce, eggs, sweetener and oil. Mix well. Blend in baking soda and flour. Add remaining ingredients; mix well. Bake in oblong pan at 350 degrees for 25 minutes or until a toothpick comes out clean. Cut into squares and put in freezer. It is good to just take out of the freezer and eat while still frozen.

DIABETIC CHOCOLATE SYRUP

1/3 c. dry cocoa
1 1/4 c. cold water
1/4 tsp. salt
2 tsp. vanilla
3 tsp. liquid sucaryl

Combine cocoa, water, and salt in a saucepan. Mix until smooth. Bring to a boil and simmer gently until smooth and thick. Allow to cool 10 minutes. Add vanilla and sweetener. Store covered in refrigerator. Stir well before using. One tablespoon equals 9 calories.

DIABETIC CREAMY FROSTING

1/2 c. low fat cottage cheese, sieved
1/8 tsp. salt
1/2 tbsp. diet margarine, melted
Non-nutritive sweetener equivalent to 1/2 c. sugar
1 tsp. almond or vanilla extract

Mix all ingredients; beat until smooth. Spread on cake. Frosts one 10 inch cake.

DIABETIC APPLESAUCE COOKIES

1/2 c. flour
1/2 tsp. baking soda
1/4 tsp. salt
1/4 tsp. nutmeg
1/2 tsp. cinnamon
1/2 c. quick cook oats
2/3 c. raisins
1/2 c. unsweet applesauce
1/4 c. vegetable oil
1 egg
1 tsp. vanilla
1 tbsp. liquid sweetener

Mix the first 6 ingredients together. Next mix the following ingredients together: Applesauce, oil, egg, vanilla and sweetener. Beat lightly. Then combine with dry ingredients and mix well together until moist. Drop on greased cookie sheet. Make sure the cookie sheet is cold. Bake at 375 degrees for 10 minutes.

DIABETIC FUDGE

1 env. gelatin
1/4 c. water
1 sq. unsweetened chocolate
1/8 tsp. cinnamon
3/4 tsp. liquid food sweetener
1/4 c. water

1/2 c. evaporated milk
1/2 tsp. vanilla
1/4 c. chopped nuts

Soften gelatin in 1/4 cup water for 5 minutes. Melt chocolate with cinnamon and sweetener; add milk and water slowly. Add gelatin. Stir until dissolved. Remove from fire. Add vanilla, cool. When mixture begins to thicken, add nuts. Turn into cold pan. When firm cut into pieces.

DIABETIC SALAD DRESSING

46 oz. low sodium V-8 juice
1 tbsp. wine vinegar
1/4 tsp. oregano
1/4 tsp. garlic powder
1/2 tsp. onion powder
1/4 packet Equal

Mix the ingredients together and chill. Shake before using.

DIABETIC COOKIES

1/2 c. Sugar Twin
1 stick margarine
1 egg
1 c. applesauce
1 c. All-Bran
1/2 tsp. allspice
1/2 tsp. nutmeg
1 tsp. soda
1 tsp. cinnamon
1 3/4 c. flour

Mix well and drop by teaspoon on cookie sheet. Bake at 350 degrees for 10 minutes.

DIABETIC PEANUT BUTTER COOKIES

1/2 c. peanut butter
2 1/2 tsp. liquid sweetener
2 eggs
1/4 tsp. baking soda
1 tbsp. butter, melted and cooled
1 c. flour
1/2 c. skim milk

Place peanut butter, butter and sweetener in mixing bowl, beat until smooth. Add eggs, beaten again. Add flour, soda and milk and mix well. Drop by teaspoon on greased cookie sheet. Bake at 375 degrees for 12-15 minutes.

DIABETIC DOUBLE CHOCOLATE COOKIES

2 c. 100% Bran or Bran Buds, All Bran or Fiber One
2/3 c. water
1 c. egg (5-6 med.)
2 tsp. vanilla
2 tsp. chocolate extract
2/3 c. vegetable oil
Liquid sugar substitute - equal to 1/2 c. sugar
1 3/4 c. flour
1/2 c. cocoa
1/4 c. dry milk (instant)
1 tsp. soda
1 tsp. baking powder

DIABETIC CHOCOLATE-NUT CANDY

1 (.75 oz.) envelope chocolate Alba 77
3 tbsp. water
1/4 c. Grape-Nut flakes
2 tbsp. chunky peanut butter
2 tbsp. raisins (optional)

Mix Alba and water together until smooth; add Grape-Nut flakes and peanut butter and raisins, if you wish. Mix well. Form into a 2x5 inch bar on aluminum foil. Wrap in foil and freeze for 2 hours. Makes 1 bar.

DIABETIC BROWNIES

1 sq. unsweetened chocolate (1 oz. melted chocolate)
2 tsp. vanilla
1 c. flour
1/4 c. chopped nuts
1/2 tsp. soda
1/2 c. shortening
2 tbsp. liquid sweetener
2 eggs
1/2 tsp. salt

DIABETIC FUDGE

1 sq. unsweetened chocolate
1/2 tsp. vanilla
1 pkg. vanilla or chocolate artificial sweetener pudding powder OR 8 tsp. finely chopped nuts
1/4 c. evaporated milk
1/4 c. chopped nuts (optional) **Don't add more nuts if used instead of the pudding powder.
1 tsp. artificial liquid sweetener

Melt chocolate and sweetener; add milk slowly. Add pudding powder or nuts. Stir until dissolved and bring to a boil. Remove from fire. Add vanilla, cool. When mixture begins to thicken, add nuts*optional. Pour into cold pan. When firm cut into squares.

DIABETIC PEACH OR STRAWBERRY JAM

1 qt. peeled peaches or 1 qt. cleanedstrawberries
2 tbsp. lemon juice
3 tsp. artificial sweetener
1 box powdered pectin

Crush peaches or strawberries in saucepan. Stir in lemon juice, pectin and sweetener. Boil 1 minute, stirring constantly. Remove from heat. Continue to stir 2 minutes. Pour into sterilized half-pint jars. Cool well. Store in the refrigerator. Yield: 2 1/2 half-pints.

DIABETIC JAM OR JELLY

2 env. unflavored gelatin
1/2 c. lemon juice
Dash of salt
1 tbsp. arrowroot
4 c. strawberries
4 c. Equal sweetener

Crush fruit and mix all ingredients together. Bring to a boil stirring constantly. Let boil for 1 minute. Remove from heat. Continue to stir for 2 minutes. Pour into sterilized jars. Cool. Store in Refrigerator.

DIABETIC LO CAL SOUR CREAM

1 c. cottage cheese
1/4 c. water
1 tbsp. lemon juice

Place all ingredients in blender. Cover and blend for 10 seconds until smooth. Makes 1 cup. Use like sour cream for dips, etc.

DIABETIC PEANUT CLUSTERS

1/3 c. peanut butter
1 tbsp. honey

1/4 c. dry roasted peanuts
1/2 c. raisins
1 tbsp. cocoa powder
1 pkt. artificial sweetener
1/4 c. Grape Nuts cereal

Melt peanut butter and honey. Remove from heat and stir in remaining ingredients except cereal. Roll rounded teaspoon of mixture into cereal to form balls. Chill and serve. Makes 12 clusters, *exchanges: 1 fruit, 1 fat, calories: 90.*

SPARKLING FRUIT DRINK - DIABETIC

8 oz. unsweetened grape juice
8 oz. unsweetened apple juice
8 oz. unsweetened orange juice
1 qt. diet ginger ale
Ice

Makes 7 servings. Mix first 4 ingredients together in a pitcher. Add ice cubes and 9 ounces of the beverage to each glass. Serve immediately. *One serving (8 oz.) = 1 fruit exchange, 60 calories.*

APPLESAUCE GELATIN SALAD FOR DIABETIC

3 (3 oz.) pkgs. raspberry Jello (sugarless)
3 c. applesauce (sugarless)
21 oz. diet 7-Up

Heat applesauce until hot. Add Jello and mix well. Add diet 7-Up blending gently. Pour into mold and refrigerate until firm.

DIABETIC GLORIFIED RICE

1/2 c. uncooked rice, not instant
1 (20 oz.) can crushed pineapple in its own juice
1 (3 oz.) pkg. sugar-free fruit flavored gelatin
1 c. boiling water

1 c. (scant) pineapple juice, drained from can
1/4 c. chopped maraschino cherries (if desired for color)
1/2 pt. heavy cream

Cook rice according to package directions. Drain and set aside. Drain pineapple, reserving 1 cup juice. Dissolve gelatin in boiling water. Add pineapple juice. Stir in well drained rice. The cooked rice will absorb the color and flavor of the gelatin. Mix well and chill until thickened, but not quite set. Add drained pineapple and cherries (if desired). Fold in cream that has been whipped. Chill. Serves 8.

DIABETIC CRANBERRY SALAD

1 pkg. frozen cranberries, put in food processor and chop finely

Add 7 packages Equal and 1 large can crushed pineapple. Set aside. 2 chopped apples 2 chopped orange sections 2 stalks chopped celery 1/2 c. nuts   Add all ingredients together and put in 9 x 12 inch dish and refrigerate.

DIABETIC COTTAGE CHEESE SALAD

1 lb. cottage cheese
1 pkg. D-Zerta dry gelatin
1 sm. can unsweetened pineapple chunks, drained
Cool Whip

Add Cool Whip to ingredients; toss lightly to mix. Serve on lettuce leaf.

DIABETIC CRANBERRY SALAD

2 pkgs. raspberry Jello or plain gelatin
1 apple
6 tsp. sweetener
2 oranges
1 lb. cranberries

Grind the oranges, apple and cranberries. Drain fruit after grinding and use the cold juice instead of water to make Jello.

DIABETIC WALDORF SALAD

4 tsp. mayonnaise
3 sm. red apples
1/4 c. chopped walnuts
2 tsp. unsweetened pineapple juice
1/2 c. diced celery

Mix mayonnaise and juice. Dice unpeeled apples. Mix with celery and walnuts. Fold in dressing. one fat exchange.

DIABETIC APRICOT SALAD

1 box apricot Jello (sugar free)
8 oz. Philly cream cheese (lite)
20 oz. can crushed pineapple (sugar-free)
Cool Whip (lite)
1/4 c. sugar (omit) (Sugar Twin, 3 pkg.)
1 c. ice water

Bring to boil crushed pineapple and sugar remove from heat and stir in Jello; then cream cheese. Add ice water, stir and let chill until getting thick. Fold in Cool Whip and chill again.

DIABETIC FRUIT SALAD

3 c. buttermilk
2 (9 oz.) boxes vanilla instant sugar free pudding mix
6 c. fresh fruit (strawberries, grapes, oranges, peaches, chunked
   pineapple, drained)
1 (8 oz.) whipped topping

Combine buttermilk and pudding in a large bowl. Fold in whipped topping. Place 1/2 the fruit mixture in an 8 x 12 Pyrex dish. Top with pudding mix. Place remaining fruit on top. People who are not diabetic enjoy this also. Recipe makes 10 generous servings.

DIABETIC CREAM OF CAULIFLOWER SOUP

4 tsp. butter or margarine
3 tbsp. flour
3/4 tsp. salt (I used none)
1/8 tsp. pepper
1 1/2 c. vegetable stock and pulp
1 1/2 c. skim milk - or exchange

 Melt butter, blend in flour, simmer on low a few minutes. Add vegetable stock and milk gradually, stirring until thickened. Use basic cream soup recipe, adding cooked pureed cauliflower, or any vegetable plus stock, saving some cauliflower florets to add when done.

DIABETIC FUDGE CAKE

1 sq. unsweetened chocolate
1/3 c. butter
2 tbsp. artificial liquid sweetener
2 tbsp. vanilla
2 eggs
1 c. cake flour
1/2 tsp. salt
1 c. walnuts

Melt butter and chocolate in saucepan over low heat. Remove from heat. Add sweetener, vanilla and eggs. Stir until well blended. Add flour, salt, soda and mix well. Fold in chopped nuts and then pour into a lightly floured and greased 9 inch square pan. Level batter and bake at 325 degrees 20-25 minutes. Cut into squares when cooled.

ORANGE NUT CAKE

1/4 c. sugar twin, brown
1/3 c. sugar twin, white
1 egg
1 1/4 c. flour
2 tsp. baking powder
1/4 tsp. soda
1/4 tsp. cinnamon
2/3 c. orange juice
1 tsp. orange extract
2 tbsp. chopped nuts

Pre-heat oven to 350 degrees. Grease 8-inch pan. In large mixing bowl, combine oleo, sugar twins, and egg. Beat 2 minutes at high speed. Scrape bowl occasionally. Lightly spoon flour into measuring cup; level off. Blend in remaining ingredients, except nuts. Beat 1 minute on slow speed. Pour mix into prepared pan. Sprinkle with nuts. Bake at 350 degrees 25 to 30 minutes.

APPLESAUCE CAKE

1 tbsp. Sweetener
1 1/2 c. unsweetened applesauce
2 tsp. Soda
1 egg
1 c. raisins
2 c. flour
1 1/2 tsp. Vanilla
1/2 c. nuts, chopped (optional)

In mixing bowl, cream oleo, sweetener, and egg. When well mixed, add applesauce, raisins, soda, and vanilla. Stir in flour. Mix well. Add nuts. Pour batter in loaf pan greased with Pam. Bake at 350 degrees 40 to 45 minutes.

DRIED FRUIT COOKIES

1/3 c. Peanut Oil
2-3 large bananas (mashed)
1 tsp. Vanilla
1/8 tsp. Salt
1 ½ c. Rolled oats
½ c. Oat Bran for hot cereal (fine cut)
1 ½ c. chopped mixed fruits (raisins, dates, apricots, peaches, etc.)
½ - ¾ c. chopped nuts

Mix peanut oil to mashed bananas. Then add vanilla, and salt. Stir in rolled oats, oat bran, chopped mixed dried fruits and chopped nuts. DROP by rounded tablespoon onto greased cookie sheets. Flatten slightly. Bake at 350 degrees for 20 to 25 minutes or until bottom and edges are lightly browned. Cool on wire rack. Store in tightly closed container in refrigerator. Makes 2 to 2 1/2 dozen.

DATE NUT MUFFINS

1 c. whole wheat flour
1 c. white flour
2 tsp. baking powder
1 tsp. cinnamon
1 1/2 tbsp. oil
1/2 c. chopped dates
1/2 c. chopped walnuts
1 egg, beaten
2 tbsp. liquid sweetener
1 c. milk

Preheat oven to 400 degrees. Mix dry ingredients. Add dates and walnuts. Make a hole in the mixture and add milk, egg, and oil. Mix until blended. Spray muffin tin with Pam and fill two thirds full. Bake for 20 to 25 minutes. Makes 12 large muffins.

NO SUGAR COOKIES

1 c. flour
1 tsp. baking powder
1/2 c. oleo
1 c. chopped nuts
1 c. flaked coconut
1/2 c. raisins
1 egg, beaten
1 c. milk
2 pkgs. Sweet 'n Low

Mix dry ingredients. Cut in oleo; stir in other ingredients. Mix until mixture sticks together and chill for 1 hour. Shape into balls. Bake at 350 degrees for 15 minutes. 48 servings.

APPLE BUTTER

2 1/4 c. sugar twin
1 tsp. nutmeg
1 tsp. cinnamon

Mix in crock pot and place 2 paper towels under lid. Cook slow for 8 hours. Makes 2 1/2 pints.

RAISIN PIE

1 1/2 c. raisins
1 1/2 c. water
1 tsp. vinegar
1/2 c. sugar twin

Boil raisins and add 3 tablespoons cornstarch in enough water to make like thin paste. Thicken raisins and pour into unbaked pie shell. Top with crust. Bake at 375 degrees until crust is done.

SUGARLESS ORANGE COOKIES

1 egg
1/2 c. oleo, softened
1/2 c. orange juice
1 tsp. grated orange rind
2 c. flour
2 tsp. baking powder
1/2 tsp. cinnamon
1/2 tsp. salt
1/2 c. chopped pecans
1/2 c. raisins

Blend egg and oleo in mixing bowl; add orange juice and orange rind, mix well. Add mixture of dry ingredients, heat until smooth. Stir in pecans and raisins; drop by spoonfuls 2 inches apart on cookie sheet. Bake at 375 degrees for 15 minutes or until brown. Yield 24 cookies.

PEANUT BUTTER SNACKS

1/2 c. peanut butter
1/2 c. honey
1 c. toasted wheat germ
2 tbsp. nonfat dry milk
1/2 c. raisins
1/2 c. coconut

Combine peanut butter, honey, wheat germ, and dry milk; mix well. Stir in raisins. Shape into balls; roll in coconut, coating well. Store covered in refrigerator. Makes 15 snacks.

DIABETIC APPLE PIE

4 c. sliced apples
1/2 c. apple juice concentrate
1 1/2 tsp. flour
1/2 tbsp. lemon juice
1 tsp. Cinnamon

Mix together. Bake in double crust at 425 degrees for 40 to 45 minutes.

DIABETIC APPLE PIE

4 c. sliced apples
1/3 cup brown sugar twin
1 Tbsp. Cinnamon
½ stick oleo or margarine

Place in unbaked pie shell. Sprinkle brown sugar twin over apples; sprinkle cinnamon on top of apples and sweetener. Slice oleo thin and place over mixture. Cover with top crust and bake at 400 degrees for 45 minutes.

PUMPKIN PIE FOR DIABETICS

2 egg whites
1 c. sugar twin
1 can pumpkin
1 can evaporated milk
Cinnamon
Nutmeg to taste

Pour into unbaked pie shell. Bake at 425 degrees for 15 minutes, then reduce heat to 350 degrees for 50 to 55 minutes or until done.

PEACH PIE FOR DIABETICS

1 can unsweetened peaches
3/4 c. sugar twin

Heat in saucepan then thicken with cornstarch. Remove from heat and add 1 teaspoon lemon juice and 1/2 teaspoon cinnamon. Pour into unbaked pie shell; top with crust. Bake at 375 degrees until crust is brown.

DIABETIC PEANUT BUTTER COOKIES

1/2 c. peanut butter
1 tbsp. butter, soft
1/3 c. brown sugar twin
2 egg whites
1 c. flour
1/4 tsp. soda
1/2 c. skim milk

Mix peanut butter, butter and sweetener. Add other ingredients, mix well. Drop by spoonfuls onto ungreased cookie sheet. Bake at 375 degrees for 12 to 15 minutes. Makes about 3 dozen.

DIABETIC CAKE

2 c. water
2 c. raisins
2 c. flour
2 eggs
3/4 c. oil
2 tbsp. liquid sweetener
1 1/4 tsp. cinnamon
1/2 tsp. nutmeg
1 tsp. soda
1 tsp. vanilla
1 c. unsweetened applesauce

Cook raising in the water until the water is gone. Add applesauce, eggs, sweetener and oil; mix well. Blend in flour and baking soda; add remaining ingredients and mix well. Bake in long flat pan at 350 degrees for about 35 minutes. (Note: I use 3 egg whites instead of eggs. This cuts down on cholesterol.)

FIG OAT BITES

1 1/2 c. flour
1/2 tsp. soda
1/4 tsp. cinnamon
1/2 c. margarine, softened
1/2 c. honey
1/4 c. skim milk
2 egg whites
2 c. Oat Bran cereal
1 c. chopped figs

Stir together flour, soda, and cinnamon. Set aside. In large mixing bowl, beat together margarine, honey, milk and egg whites. Add flour mixture, stirring until combined. Mix cereal and figs; drop by tablespoon onto lightly greased baking sheet. Flatten slightly with bottom of floured glass. Bake at 375 degrees for about 10 minutes or until lightly browned. Yield 3 dozen cookies. 2 cookies = 170 calories

----

MOLTED VEGETABLE SALAD

1 pkg. sugar-free lemon Jello
2 c. boiling water
2 tbsp. lemon juice
2/3 c. cabbage, chopped
2/3 c. green pepper, chopped
2 slices pimiento
Lettuce leaves

Dissolve gelatin in boiling water and stir until completely dissolved. Add lemon juice, add chopped vegetables and chill. Slice when firm and serve on lettuce leaves with low-calorie dressing. This recipe may be a free food. It is 20 calories and has large amounts of vitamins A and C.

JELLO SALAD

1 box sugar-free Jello, any flavor
8 oz. sour cream
8 oz. Cool Whip
8 oz. crushed pineapple

Mix well Jello, sour cream and pineapple. Fold in Cool Whip and chill.
Serves 8.

PINEAPPLE FLUFF

2 c. unsweetened pineapple with juice
1 1/3 c. non-fat dry milk
3 pkgs. Equal
3 tbsp. lemon juice
1 tsp. vanilla
1 tsp. butter-flavoring
1 pkg. lemon or lime gelatin

Dissolve gelatin in 1/2 cup boiling water. Put pineapple, dry milk,
sugar substitute, lemon juice, vanilla, and butter flavoring in blender
and blend 1 minute, scraping sides. Add gelatin and blend 3 more
minutes, until foamy. Pour into a square dish and refrigerate.   4
servings.

PEAR BREAD

3 c. flour
1 tsp. soda
1/4 tsp. baking powder
1 tsp. salt (optional)
1 tbsp. cinnamon
1 c. chopped pecans
3/4 c. vegetable oil
3 eggs, slightly beaten
2 c. sugar (substitute 18 pkgs. Sweet & Low or Sugar Twin)
2 c. peeled, grated pears
2 tsp. vanilla

Combine first six ingredients in large bowl. Make a well in center and add oil, eggs, sugar, pears and vanilla. Stir just until moist. Put into 2 greased loaf pans. Bake at 325 degrees for 1 hour and 15 minutes or until tests done.

PUMPKIN BREAD

1 c. shortening
1 (#303) can pumpkin
3 1/2 c. flour
1/2 tsp. baking powder
1 tsp. cinnamon
1 tsp. cloves
1 tsp. allspice
3 eggs
1/2 c. plus 2 tbsp. Sweet & Low or Sugar Twin
1 tsp. baking soda
1 tsp. nutmeg
1/2 c. chopped nuts

Mix shortening, eggs and pumpkin. In separate bowl combine dry ingredients and add to pumpkin mixture and blend well. Add nuts and stir. Pour into 2 greased and floured loaf pans and bake at 325 degrees for 1 hour. Let cool before removing from pans.

APPLESAUCE BRAN MUFFINS

1 c. Bran Buds or 100% Bran
1/4 c. vegetable oil
1 egg
1 c. unsweetened applesauce
Liquid sugar substitute equal to ¼ c. sugar (optional)
2 tbsp. brown sugar
2 tbsp. water
1 c. all-purpose flour
1 tsp. soda
2 tbsp. dry buttermilk
1/2 tsp. salt
1 tsp. cinnamon

Mix together bran, egg, oil, applesauce, sugar substitute, brown sugar, and water, let set at room temperature for 30-45 minutes. Stir together flour, soda, dry buttermilk, salt and cinnamon. Add to bran mixture and mix at medium speed only until flour is moistened. Spray muffin tins with Pam, or line them with paper liners. Fill about 1/2 full and bake at 400 degrees for 20 minutes or until they spring back when touched in center. Serve hot. Makes 12 muffins.

SWEET FREE PEACH PIE

1 1/2 c. concentrated or 12 oz. can apple juice
3 tbsp. cornstarch
1 oz. butter or margarine
1/2 tsp. cinnamon
6 pkgs. Equal sweetener
4 c. fresh or frozen peaches
Unbaked pie shell

Cookl until butter melts all ingredients. Pour in pie shell and bake at 350 degrees for 45 minutes.

SUGAR-FREE STRAWBERRY PIE

1 baked pie crust
Fresh strawberries
1 box sugar-free strawberry Jello
Cool Whip
Bake pie crust for about 10 minutes at 400 degrees. Cool and layer with fresh strawberries. Mix Jello. When cool, pour Jello over strawberries. Chill until set. Cover with Cool Whip.

OATMEAL COOKIES

1 1/2 c. quick cooking oatmeal, uncooked
2/3 c. melted butter
2 eggs, beaten
1 tbsp. liquid sweetener
1 1/2 c. sifted cake flour

1/2 tsp. salt
2 tsp. baking powder
1/2 c. skim milk
1 tsp. vanilla
1/4 c. raisins
1/4 c. nuts, if desired

Measure oatmeal into mixing bowl, stir in melted butter and mix well. Blend in eggs and sweetener. Add dry ingredients alternately with milk and vanilla, add raisins and nuts. Drop by teaspoon on cookie sheet. Bake at 400 degrees for 10 to 15 minutes or until golden brown. Makes about 72 cookies. *Exchange 2 cookies for 1/2 of bread and 1/4 fat – calories(2 cookies)= 63.*

RAISIN CAKE

2 c. water
1 c. unsweetened applesauce
1/2 tsp. nutmeg
2 eggs
2 c. flour
1/2 tsp. salt
2 tbsp. liquid sweetener
1 tsp. soda
1 3/4 tsp. cinnamon
2 c. raisins
3/4 c. cooking oil
1 tsp. vanilla

Cook water and raisins until water is gone. Add applesauce, eggs, liquid sweetener, blend in cooking oil, soda, flour, nutmeg, and cinnamon and salt. Pour into greased tube pan and bake 25 minutes. Good when served hot. Bake at 325 degrees.

DATE COFFEE CAKE

1/3 c. mashed ripe bananas
1/2 c. butter, softened
3 lg. eggs
1 1/4 c. water

1 1/2 c. chopped dates
1 tsp. vanilla
2 tsp. baking powder
1 tsp. baking soda
3 c. unbleached white flour

Beat together mashed bananas and butter until creamy, add eggs, vanilla and water, beat. Measure in flour, baking soda and baking powder, beat well stir in dates. Spoon batter into oiled and floured 9 x 13 inch baking pan and spread evenly.
--TOPPING--
1/3 c. chopped dates
1/3 c. chopped walnuts
1/3 c. flaked coconut

Combine these three and sprinkle over batter. Bake at 350 degrees for 20 to 25 minutes or until inserted knife comes out clean. Cool on rack 8 to 10 minutes.

DATE NUT CAKE

1 stick margarine
1 egg
1 tsp. vanilla
1 tbsp. liquid sweetener
1 1/2 c. unsweetened applesauce
1 c. chopped dates
1 c. pecans
2 c. flour
1/2 tsp. cinnamon
1/4 tsp. cloves
2 tsp. soda

Mix together margarine, egg, vanilla, sweetener and applesauce. Stir in dates and pecans. Sift together dry ingredients and add to mixture mixing well. Bake in loaf pan at 350 degrees for 1 hour.

DARK BRAN MUFFINS

1 c. all-purpose flour
1 tsp. baking soda
1 c. all bran, bran or 100% bran
2 lg. egg whites at room temperature
Liquid sugar substitute equal to 3 tbsp. sugar
1 c. water
2 tbsp. vegetable oil
1/4 c. dark molasses
1/4 c. dry buttermilk

Place flour, soda, bran and dry buttermilk in mixer bowl and mix at low speed to blend. Combine water, egg whites, oils, sweetener, and molasses and stir with a fork until moistened. Grease muffin tins with margarine or line with paper liners. Fill muffin tin half full and bake at 400 degrees for 20 to 25 minutes, or until muffins spring back when touched in the center. *97 calories, 16 grams cholesterol, 3 grams protein, 3 grams fat, NA 154 milligrams. Food exchanges per serving, 1 bread, 1/2 fat.*

BAKED BEANS

1 lb. dry great northern beans
4 oz. chopped center cut ham
6 oz. tomato paste
2 tbsp. salad mustard
Cold water as necessary
1 c. chopped onions
1 1/2 tsp. salt
3/4 c. Brown Sugar Twin

Wash beans, add cold water to cover, bring to a boil. Simmer for 5 minutes. Remove from heat, and let stand 2 to 3 hours. Drain well. Cover again with cold water to about 1/2 inch over top of beans. Bring to a boil, reduce heat, cover and let simmer for about 2 1/2 hours or until the beans are soft. Mix beans and remaining ingredients. Place in shallow baking dish and bake uncovered at 325 degrees for 2 to 3 hours stirring every hour. *1/3 cup serving - calories 115. cholesterol 18 grams, protein 7 grams, fat 2 grams, NA 262 milligrams. Food exchange, 1 bread, 1 lean meat, Omit salt for low sodium diets.*

CHOCOLATE SAUCE

3 tbsp. cocoa
4 tsp. cornstarch
1/3 c. instant dry milk
10 (1 gram) pkg. Equal
1/8 tsp. salt
1 tbsp. margarine
2 tsp. vanilla

Stir cocoa, cornstarch, dry milk and salt to blend in a small saucepan. Stir water into dry mixture until smooth. Add margarine and cook and stir over low heat. Bring to a boil and simmer for 2 minutes, stirring constantly. Remove from heat. Add vanilla and sweetener to sauce. Stir lightly to mix. Pour into a glass jar and refrigerate until used. Return to room temperature before serving over ice cream or it may be heated gain to serve over cake or pudding. 2 tablespoons per serving. *Calories 31, cholesterol 3 grams, protein 1 gram, fat 2 grams, NA 52 milligrams. Food exchanges per serving, 1/2 vegetable. Low sodium diets - omit salt.*

MAYONNAISE

1/2 tsp. dry mustard
Juice of 1 lemon
3/4 c. unsaturated oil
1 tsp. salt
1 egg

Put first 4 ingredients into a bowl and beat until smooth. Add oil 1 tablespoon at a time for about 5 additions. Beat well after each addition. Pour remaining oil in a thin stream, beating constantly. Makes approximately 1 cup. One teaspoon contains 3 grams fat and 30 calories. Exchange value 2 teaspoons, 1 fat exchange.

SWISS STEAK

1 lb. round steak

2 tsp. vinegar
Seasonings to taste
2 med. onions, sliced
1/2 c. celery, diced

Trim round steak and portion into 4 equal parts. Pound to break down tissue. Sear meat on both sides. Cover with water, add vinegar, onion, celery, and seasonings. Continue cooking in oven or on stove until tender. Two cups tomato juice may be used in place of water. Exchange 1 serving: 3 meat exchanges.

BEEF STEW

1 lb. lean cubed beef
2 bay leaves
4 sm. potatoes, peeled & cubed
1/4 c. sliced onions
6 sm. whole carrots

Cube beef in 1 1/2 inch cubes, sear on all sides. Cover meat with boiling water, add onions and bay leaves. Cover pot and simmer for 1 1/2 hours. Add vegetables and cook another 30 minutes.

MEAT LOAF

1 lb. lean ground beef
1 tbsp. chopped onion
1/4 tsp. Worcestershire sauce
1/2 tsp. artificial liquid sweetener
2 tbsp. minced green pepper
1 1/2 c. tomato juice
1/2 tsp. salt
1/4 tsp. pepper

Mix ingredients and mold into a loaf pan. Bake in a moderate oven (375 degrees) for 30 to 45 minutes. Yield: 4 servings. Exchange: 1 serving for 3 meat exchanges and 1 vegetable exchange.

BAKED FISH FILLETS

1 lb. fish fillets
1/2 tsp. salt (optional)
4 tsp. liquid margarine
1/4 c. skim milk
4 tbsp. fine dry bread crumbs

Cut fillets into four portions and soak 3 minutes in milk. Drain and roll in bread crumbs. Place fish on a greased baking dish. Bake in a very hot oven (450 to 475 degrees), allow 8 minutes if fish is fresh and 15 minutes if fish is frozen, or until fish flakes easily with a fork. Yield: 4 servings. Exchange: 1 serving for 3 meat exchanges and 1/2 bread exchange and 1 fat exchange.

STUFFED GREEN PEPPER

1 sm. green pepper
3 level tbsp. cooked & drained rice
Salt & pepper to taste
1 tsp. chopped onion
1 tsp. chopped celery
1/3 c. tomato juice

Wash and cut stem end from green pepper and remove seeds and membrane. Place in pan with ½" to 1 " water in bottom. Mix cooked rice, chopped onion, celery, salt, pepper and tomato juice together. Fill green pepper with rice mixture. Bake in a moderate oven 350 to 375 degrees basting frequently until onions are tender, about 30 minutes. *1 serving per green pepper. Exchange for 1 vegetable exchange and 1 bread exchange.*

VEGETABLE SOUP

3 c. soup stock
1/4 c. chopped onions
1/4 c. green beans cut in strips
2 tbsp. diced turnip
1/4 c. diced carrots
1/4 c. shredded cabbage

1 tbsp. celery, finely chopped
Salt, pepper, seasoning

Add prepared vegetables to soup stock. Cook until vegetables are tender (about 1/2 hour). Season to taste. Serve hot. *NOTE:* Any combination of vegetables may be used in this recipe, as long as their exchange value adds up to one vegetable exchange. *Exchange 1 serving for 1 vegetable serving.*

BAKED TOMATOE

1 med. sized tomatoe
Other seasonings to taste
1/2 tsp. chopped parsley
Salt & pepper
1/2 tsp. chopped onion
1/2 tsp. sage or chives

Wash tomatoe and cut out stem end. Place in small baking dish with a little water in the bottom, about 1/2 inch. Sprinkle with seasonings of choice. Bake in a moderate oven (350 degrees) until tomato is tender but not so soft it will fall apart. About 15 to 20 minutes. Yield 1 serving. Exchange for 1 vegetable exchange.

SPICED POT ROAST

2 lb. boneless chuck beef
1 bay leaf
Salt, pepper, vinegar, water
1 med. onion, sliced
1 tsp. whole pepper berries

Rub meat with salt and pepper and place in glass bowl. Add onion, bay leaf, and whole pepper berries, marinate meat in equal parts vinegar and water for 24 hours. Drain and reserve liquid. Place meat in roasting pan, sear well. Add 3 tablespoons spiced vinegar mixture. Cover and cook in slow oven for 1 1/2 hours. 8 servings. *Exchange one 3-ounce serving or 3 slices each measuring 4 x 2 x 1/4 inches for 3 meat exchanges.*

HOT DOG DELIGHT

1 wiener, cooked
1 slice pre-sliced processed cheese
1 strip partially cooked bacon
1 wiener roll

Roll cheese around wiener which has been cooked, and roll the partially cooked bacon around both cheese and wiener. Fasten with toothpicks. Broil for 1 or 2 minutes. Place on heated wiener bun. 1 serving. *Exchange for 2 meat exchange, 1 fat exchange and 2 bread exchanges.*

COTTAGE CHEESE VEGETABLE DUNK

2 (8 ounce) cartons low fat cottage cheese
1 cup (4 ounce) shredded low fat process American cheese
3 tablespoons plain unsweetened low fat yogurt,
2 tablespoons prepared horseradish
1/2 teaspoon pepper
1/4 teaspoon salt
2 tablespoons chopped green pepper
2 tablespoons minced onion

Mix cottage cheese, american cheese, yogurt, horseradish, pepper, salt, green pepper, and minced onion. 28 servings. *Exchange free. Calories 22, trace of fat, cholesterol 1 milligram, carbohydrate 1 gram, trace of fiber, protein 3 milligrams, sodium 134 milligrams.*

COLE SLAW

1 tbsp. finely chopped onion
1 tbsp. low fat mayonnaise
2 c. finely shredded cabbage
2 tsp. prepared mustard
1/4 tsp. salt
Toasted sesame seeds

Mix dressing ingredients and toss with cabbage. Garnish with toasted sesame seeds (or wheat germ). 4 servings. *Total recipe contains 11 grams carbohydrate, 4 grams protein and 0 grams fat. One serving (1/2 cup) contains 3 grams carbohydrate and vitamin C. Exchange value 1 group A vegetable.*

APPLESAUCE BRAN SQUARES

1 c. all-purpose flour
1 tsp. cinnamon
1/4 tsp. cloves or nutmeg
1/2 c. oleo (room temperature)
2 lg. egg whites (room temperature)
1 tsp. vanilla
Liquid sugar equal to 1/2 c. sugar
2/3 c. bran buds
1/2 c. rolled oats
2 tbsp. brown sugar
1/2 tsp. salt
1/2 tsp. baking soda
1/3 c. chopped nuts
1 c. unsweetened applesauce

Place dry ingredients in mixer bowl and mix at low speed for 1 minute. Add oleo, egg whites, vanilla, sugar substitute, nuts, and applesauce to flour mixture and mix at medium speed for 1 minute or until blended. Spread evenly in a 9 x 13 cake pan which has been greased with oleo or sprayed with PAM spray. Bake at 375 degrees for 25 to 30 minutes or until browned and it starts to pull away from the sides of pan. Cut into 3 x 5 squares and serve warm or room temperature. *One square per serving. Calories 135, cholesterol 14 milligrams, fat 8 grams, NA 24 milligrams, 1 bread and 1 1/2 fat.*

ZERO SALAD DRESSING

1/2 c. tomato juice
1 tbsp. onion, finely chopped
2 tbsp. lemon juice or vinegar
Salt & pepper to taste

Chopped parsley or green pepper, horseradish or mustard may be added if desired. Combine ingredients in a jar with a tightly fitted top. Shake well before using. Use as desired.

SUGAR - FREE APPLE PIE

4 c. sliced peeled apples
1/2 c. frozen apple juice concentrate
1 tsp. cinnamon or apple pie spice
1/2 tsp. lemon juice, optional
2 tsp. tapioca or cornstarch

Mix apples, apple juice concentrate, thickener and spice and stir until apples are well-coated, add lemon juice, if desired, to keep apples lighter colored. Taste 1 piece of apple to check the spice. Pour into the pastry lined pie pan and top with the second crust or pastry strips. Seal the edges and cut slits in the top crust to allow steam to escape. Bake at 425 degrees for 40 to 45 minutes, or until golden brown. Serve warm or cold.

LEMON SAUCE

2 c. water
2 tbsp. cornstarch
1/8 tsp. salt
Grated rind of 1 lemon
2 tbsp. margarine
2 tbsp. lemon juice
1 drop yellow food coloring
8 (1 gram) pkg. Equal

Combine water, cornstarch, and salt. Stir until smooth in a small saucepan. Cook and stir over medium heat until thickened and clear, then continue to simmer, stirring constantly for another 2 minutes. Remove from heat and add remaining ingredients to sauce, stir lightly to mix well. Serve warm over cake or pudding. 1/4 cup per serving. 38 calories, 3 grams cholesterol, nege grams protein, 3 milligrams fat, 68 milligrams NA. 1/2 fat, 1/2 vegetable exchanges.

PEANUT BUTTER COOKIES

1/2 cup chunky peanut butter
1/3 cup oleo (both at room temperature
1/4 cup dark molasses
2 teaspoons liquid sugar substitute
1 1/4 c. all-purpose flour
12 teaspoon baking soda
18 teaspoon salt

Cream together at medium speed until smooth:
peanut butter, oleo (both at room temperature), sugar substitute. Set aside. Then sift flour, baking soda, and salt together. Add to creamed mixture, mix at medium speed until smooth. Drop by tablespoon onto cookie sheet lined with foil. Press down lightly with fingers dipped in cold water to form circles 2-inches wide. Bake at 375 degrees for 10 to 12 minutes or until lightly browned. Remove to wire rack. *2 cookies per serving. 140 calories, 13 grams cholesterol, 4 grams protein, 9 gram fat, 169 milligrams NA. 1 bread and 2 fat exchanges.*

FRUIT MILKSHAKE

 Place the following in the blender: 1/2 c. papaya juice
1/3 c. old-fashioned oatmeal
1 tbsp. non-fat powdered milk
2 env. Equal
1/2 c. frozen fruit strawberries, raspberries, blackberries, blueberries)
    and unsweetened applesauce mixed, OR 1/2 banana
2 tbsp. frozen orange juice, not diluted
1/2 c. milk (2% or less)
1 tsp. vanilla

Blend, pour into large glass and ENJOY!

FRUIT AND SPICE COOKIES

2 cups dates
1 1/2 cups raisins

3 eggs (or 1/2 carton of Eggbeaters)
2 1/2 cups flour
1/2 pound oleo
1/4 cup sugar
1/4 cup sugar substitute + 2 heaping tsp. more sugar substitute
1/4 tsp. allspice
1/2 tsp. salt
1 1/2 c. quick cooking oatmeal
1/3 c. oil
1/4 tsp. cloves
1 1/2 tsp. cinnamon
2 tsp. soda
2 tsp. Vanilla
1 tsp. Nutmeg

Mix together dates, raisins. Then add eggs. Let soak. Mix like pie crust: flour, oleo, sugar, sugar substitute. Use generous measures for spices:

Mix remainng ingredients together until well blended. Add fruit and egg mixture and blend. May also add 1/2 to 1 cup crushed, undrained pineapple, if desired. Drop from spoon on lightly greased cookie sheet. Bake at 375 degrees for 10 minutes. Makes about 5 dozen.

GINGERBREAD

1 c. unsifted flour
1/2 tsp. baking soda
1/4 tsp. salt
1/2 tsp. cinnamon
1/2 tsp. ginger
3 tbsp. butter
1 egg
1/2 c. molasses
6 tbsp. boiling water

Combine flour, soda, salt, cinnamon, and ginger, mixing well; set aside. Cream butter until fluffy, add egg and molasses, blending well. Add dry ingredients, alternately with water. Turn into greased 8 inch baking pan. Bake in 325 degree oven for about 25 minutes or until done. Makes 12 servings. 102 calories per serving.

JELLO COTTAGE CHEESE SALAD

1 (3 1/2 oz.) pkg. lime Jello
1 (3 1/2 oz.) pkg. lemon Jello
3 c. water and pineapple juice, boiling
1 (8 1/2 oz.) can crushed pineapple
1 can standard evaporated milk
1 c. mayonnaise
1 c. cottage cheese

Mix all ingredients together and enjoy!

LOW-CALORIE BROWNIES

2 c. fine graham cracker crumbs, (28 crackers)
1/2 tsp. cinnamon
1/4 tsp. salt
1 c. skim milk
1 tsp. vanilla
1/2 c. semi-sweet chocolate pieces, melted
1/2 c. chopped nuts
1 tbsp. sifted powdered sugar

Combine crumbs, cinnamon and salt. Stir in milk and vanilla, mixing well. Add chocolate and nuts; blend thoroughly. Turn into lightly greased 9 inch pan. Bake in 350 degree preheated oven for 15 to 20 minutes, or just until done. Turn out on rack to cool. Cut into 40 pieces; sprinkle powdered sugar over top. 44 calories per piece.

MOLDED HOLIDAY SALAD

1 lg. pkg. sugar free strawberry or cherry Jello
1 pkg. CONDENSED mincemeat

Dissolve Jello in two cups boiling water. Add one cup cold water. Cool. Crumble mincemeat in 1 1/4 cups water. Place pan on heat and bring to boil, stirring, and cook until thickened. Let cool. Add to the cooled Jello and pour into a shallow pan and refrigerate. When set, cut into squares, place on lettuce leaf and serve with either mayonnaise or Cool Whip.

ORANGE-PINEAPPLE MOLD

1 (No. 2) can crushed pineapple, in unsweetened pineapple juice
2 env. unflavored gelatin
1/4 c. sugar
1/4 tsp. salt
1 c. unsweetened pineapple juice (from crushed pineapple)
3 eggs, separated
1 c. fresh orange juice
1 c. buttermilk
1 tsp. grated lemon rind
1 tsp. grated orange rind

Drain pineapple, reserving juice. Combine gelatin, sugar and salt in saucepan. Add small amount of pineapple juice to make smooth paste. Add egg yolks and blend well. Add remaining pineapple juice. Cook, stirring, over medium heat until gelatin is dissolved and mixture coats a spoon. DO NOT BOIL. Remove from heat and cool to lukewarm, stirring occasionally. Add orange juice, buttermilk, lemon, and orange rind; blend thoroughly. Cool until mixture starts to thicken. Beat egg whites until stiff; fold into gelatin mixture along with 1 cup of the drained pineapple. Turn into 6 cup mold. Chill several hours until set. Unmold on serving plate and garnish as desired. Makes 8 servings. 119 calories per serving.

PINEAPPLE-CHEESE PIE

1 (24 oz.) carton cottage cheese
1 pkg. Knox gelatin
1 egg
1 sm. can crushed pineapple
3 pkgs. Sweet & Low
2 tsp. vanilla
2 tsp. lemon juice
1 tsp. rum flavor
Cinnamon

Process cottage cheese until smooth and set aside. Drain pineapple juice in bowl, add Knox gelatin and set aside for five minutes. To cottage cheese add egg, Sweet & Low, lemon juice and flavorings. Blend well. Add pineapple juice mixture and blend again. Stir

pineapple into cheese mixture. Pour into an 8 inch or 9 inch pie plate and sprinkle with cinnamon. Bake 30 minutes in 350 degree oven. Cool and set in refrigerator overnight.TOPPING:
1 (15 oz.) can crushed pineapple, drained
1 pkg. Sweet & Low
1 tsp. cornstarch
1 tsp. rum flavoring

To drained pineapple juice, add Sweet & Low and cornstarch. Cook on medium heat, stirring, until mixture is smooth and thick. Add crushed pineapple and rum flavoring. Cool and serve on pie.

PINEAPPLE SALAD

1 pkg. lemon or lime low-calorie gelatin dessert
1 c. boiling water
1 (8 oz.) can crushed pineapple in unsweetened pineapple juice
1/2 of a 12 oz. can citrus or lemon-lime sugar-free carbonated beverage
4 oz. whipped topping (about1/2 of an 8 oz. container)

RICE KRISPIES COOKIES

1/4 c. brown sugar
1/4 c. sugar substitute plus 2 heaping tsp. of sugar substitute (16 env. of Weight Watchers sugar substitute)
1/2 lb. oleo

Mix well. 1 cup of oil add to 3 eggs (or use 1/2 of Eggbeaters), 2 teaspoons vanilla. Mix in dry ingredients and blend well.

Mix dry ingredients together first:
3 1/2 c. flour
1 tsp. baking powder
1 tsp. cream of tartar
1/2 tsp. salt
1 c. quick cooking oatmeal
1 1/2 c. Rice Krispies
3/4 c. nuts

STRAWBERRY RHUBARB SALAD

2 c. cooked rhubarb (sweetened to taste)
1 pkg. strawberry gelatin
1/2 c. finely chopped nuts
1/2 c. finely chopped celery
1 (3 oz.) pkg. cream cheese, softened

Mix all ingredients together well.

SUGARLESS BARS

3 bananas, mashed
2 eggs
1/3 c. Saffola
1 c. buttermilk
1 c. flour
2 tsp. cinnamon
1 tsp. nutmeg
1 tsp. cloves
1 tsp. allspice
1 tsp. soda
2 c. old-fashioned rolled oats
1 tsp. vanilla
1 c. chopped dates
1/2 c. chopped nuts

Combine flour, and spices, mixing well; set aside. Cream bananas, eggs, saffola, buttermilk, and vanilla, blending well. Add dry ingredients, then add dates, nuts and oats. Pout into greased 9x13 inch baking pan. Bake in 325 degree oven for about 25 minutes or until done.

SWEETBREADS AND MUSHROOMS

1 lb. sweetbreads
3 c. water
1 tbsp. vinegar
2 tsp. salt (seasoned)
1 1/2 tbsp. butter

2/3 c. chopped green onion
2 c. sliced fresh mushrooms
1/8 tsp. thyme
1/2 c. sherry

Wash sweetbreads and soak in cold water for 20 minutes. Drain and add the 3 cups water, vinegar, and 1 teaspoon of the salt. Bring to a boil; cover and simmer for 20 minutes until tender. Let cool in liquid for 20 minutes. Drain; remove membranes and dice sweetbreads; set aside. Melt butter in non-stick skillet. add onion and saute for 5 minutes. Add mushrooms and saute 5 minutes longer. Sprinkle on remaining salt and thyme. Add sweetbreads and sherry. Cover and simmer until thoroughly heated. Serve immediately. Makes 6 servings. 130 calories per serving.

THOUSAND ISLAND DRESSING

Stir together:2 c. plain yogurt
2 hard-cooked eggs, minced
Enough catsup to make a coral color

Variations - Add one or two envelopes of Equal if a sweeter dressing is desired. Use steak sauce if a sharper flavor suits you better.

VEAL SCALLOPINI

1 1/2 lbs. veal, round or loin
2 tbsp. flour
1 1/2 tsp. seasoned salt
Dash pepper
1 tbsp. butter
2 c. sliced, fresh mushrooms
1/4 c. beef broth
2 tbsp. dry sherry

Trim meat well and cut into 6 pieces. Combine flour, salt, and pepper; sprinkle onto both sides of veal. Melt butter in non-stick skillet; add meat and brown quickly on either side; transfer to hot serving platter to keep warm. Add mushrooms and saute about 5 minutes; add beef broth and sherry. Cook over high heat for about 1 minute. Serve over veal. Makes 6 servings. 252 calories per serving.

LOW-CALORIE TOMATO DRESSING

1 c. tomato juice
1/4 c. salad oil
1/4 c. vinegar
1 tsp. salt
1 tsp. dry mustard
1/4 tsp. garlic salt
1/4 tsp. onion salt
1 tbsp. steak sauce

Combine all ingredients and beat well to mix thoroughly. Chill. Good on salad greens. Makes 1 1/2 cups. Total calories: 458; 19 calories per tablespoon.

LOW CALORIE SALAD DRESSING

1/2 c. cottage cheese
1/2 c. buttermilk
1/2 lemon, peeled and seeded
1 tsp. salt
1/2 tsp. paprika
1/2 green pepper
4 radishes
Dash of salt

Put all the ingredients in a blender and blend until the green pepper and the radishes are finely chopped.

YOGURT SALAD DRESSING

2 c. yogurt
3-4 tbsp. soy sauce
1/4 c. toasted sesame seeds
2 tbsp. celery seeds

2 tbsp. dill weed
1 tbsp. onion, chopped

Combine ingredients and blend in blender.

PINEAPPLE SALAD DRESSING

1 c. pineapple juice
1/2 c. sugar
1 tbsp. cornstarch
1 egg white, beaten
Pinch of salt
2 tbsp. lemon juice
1/4 tsp. grated lemon rind

Cook pineapple juice, cornstarch and salt until thickened. Fold in stiffly beaten egg white last. Whipping cream can be added if a richer dressing is desired.

UNSALTED CHICKEN

Place chicken pieces in oiled baking dish. Sprinkle on chicken:
2 tsp. minced garlic
Grated lemon rind
Juice of 1/2 lemon
Thyme and oregano
2 tbsp. water or unsalted broth
Sprinkle of oil

Bake in oven for about 30 min (or until golden brown) at 350 degrees.

OVEN BEEF STEW

2 lbs. beef stew meat, lean
2 med. onions, chopped
1 c. cut celery
2 c. (or more) sliced carrots
3 or 4 med. potatoes, chunked
2 heaping tbsp. tapioca

1 tbsp. sugar
1 tbsp. salt
About 2 c. tomato juice

Put in large casserole or roaster with tight cover. Sprinkle with
chopped parsley, cover and bake at 250 degrees for 5 to 7 hours. May
omit salt for salt free diet.

BAKED FISH

Any fish fillet
1/4 c. margarine
1 tbsp. lemon juice
1/4 tsp. freshly ground pepper
1/4 tsp. basil

Melt margarine add lemon juice, pepper and basil. Dip fillets in
mixture and then in dry bread crumbs. Lay in one layer in greased
pan. Bake at 400 degrees for 15 minutes or until done. Good for no
salt, low cholesterol diet.

DIABETIC FRUIT BARS

--FRUIT MIXTURE--
1/2 c. raisins
1/2 c. chopped prunes
1 c. water

Boil fruit together for 5 minutes. Add 1/2 cup butter or margarine, set
aside to cool.
--BATTER--
2 eggs, beaten
1 tsp. soda
1 tsp. vanilla
1/4 tsp. salt
1/2 tsp. cinnamon
1/4 tsp. nutmeg
1 c. flour
1/2 c. chopped nuts

Add batter to fruit mixture. Bake in an 11"x7" greased pan at 350 degrees for 25 to 30 minutes. Cool and cut.

NO SALT DRY SOUP MIX

2 c. non-fat dry milk
3/4 c. cornstarch
1/4 c. instant chicken bouillon
2 tbsp. dry onion flakes
1 tsp. thyme
1 tsp. basil
1/8 tsp. pepper

Use 1/3 cup mix to 1 cup boiling water. May add vegetables. Whole kernel corn, leftover meat.

EGG SUBSTITUTE

1 tbsp. dry milk
2 egg whites, from lg. eggs
2 tsp. corn oil
4 drops yellow food coloring
Sm. bowl

Sprinkle powdered milk over egg whites and oil beat with fork add coloring beat until smooth. Makes 1 egg.

DIABETIC DATE BARS

Night Before: Mix 1 cup chopped dates, 1 1/2 cups applesauce (unsweetened). Cut up dates into applesauce. Add 3 to 4 packets of equal, refrigerate overnight. 1 tsp. vanilla 1/2 c. margarine, melted 2 c. flour 2 tsp. soda 1/4 tsp. cloves 1/2 tsp. cinnamon   Mix dry ingredients. Add beaten eggs, margarine and vanilla. Add date mixture last. Pour into 9"x13" pan. Sprinkle with 1/2 cup chopped pecans. Bake at 350 degrees for 30 minutes.

MEAT LOAF

Altered for low salt, no sugar, low cholesterol diet. 1/2 c. dry bread crumbs 1/4 c. dried milk 1/2 c. water 1/4 c. chopped green pepper 1 med. onion, chopped 2 egg whites 1/4 c. low sodium catsup 2 tsp. prepared horseradish 1 tsp. prepared mustard   Combine ingredients; mix well. Pack in 9"x5" loaf pan or 2 small pans. Spread with Topping:
--TOPPING--
3 tbsp. brown Sugar Twin
1/4 c. light low sodium catsup
1/4 tsp. nutmeg
1 tsp. dry mustard

Blend all ingredients. If made in 2 small pans, one may be frozen. Bake 45 minutes at 375 degrees.

SWEET 'N SOUR CHICKEN

1/2 c. chopped green pepper
1/2 c. chopped carrots
1/2 c. chopped onion
3/4 c. lite catsup
2 tbsp. Vinegar
2 tbsp. low sodium soy sauce
1 c. pineapple juice
1/4 c. brown Sugar Twin
1/2 tsp. garlic powder
1/4 tsp. freshly ground pepper
Dash ground ginger
1 c. pineapple chunks, drained

Heat margarine in large skillet until melted. Add green pepper, carrots and onion. Cook and stir 5 minutes. Add catsup, pineapple juice, vinegar, soy sauce, Sugar Twin, garlic powder, pepper and ginger. Cook, stirring, until it boils. Add pineapple chunks. Arrange skinned chicken parts (about 3 lbs.) in 9"x13" pan. Pour sauce over all. Cover tightly with foil. Bake 45 minutes in 400 degree oven. Uncover and bake 30 minutes or until done. Serve with rice. Good recipe for those on a no salt, no sugar, low cholesterol diet.

CLUB TURKEY CASSEROLE

1/4 c. margarine
1/3 c. flour
1 c. turkey*
2 c. skim milk
1 1/2 tsp. salt
1/2 c. blanched almonds, slivered & toasted
1 c. brown rice, cook & should yield 4 c.
2 1/2 c. diced, cooked turkey
1 (3 or 4 oz.) can mushrooms, drained
1/2 c. chopped pimiento
1/3 c. chopped green pepper

  *Or chicken broth made with 2 teaspoons chicken bouillon in 1 cup water. Cook rice. In a large size pan, melt margarine, blend in flour. Stir in broth and milk. Cook over low heat until thickened, stirring constantly. Stir in remaining ingredients except almonds. Pour into spray treated 9"x13" pan. Top with almonds and bake at 350 degrees, uncovered. May omit salt for no salt low cholesterol diet.

CARROT SALAD

1 1/2 c. grated carrots
1 c. raisins
1/2 c. sliced celery
1/2 c. chopped nuts
1/3 c. mayonnaise
1/4 tsp. salt (opt.)

Combine ingredients and chill. (Can use "light", no cholesterol mayonnaise.)

RHUBARB BARS

1 1/2 c. sugar
2 tbsp. Cornstarch
1/4 c. water

1 teaspoon vanilla
1 1/2 c. flour
1 c. brown sugar
1/2 tsp. Soda
1 c. soft butter or margarine
1/2 c. chopped walnuts

Mix sugar,cornstarch, and water, cook until thick. Add vanilla. Mix flour, sugar, soda, butter, and nuts until crumbly: Pat about 2/3 of crumb mixture in 9"x13" pan. Pour over the rhubarb mixture. Top with remaining crumbs. Bake 30 to 35 minutes at 375 degrees.

GAZPACHO

4 tomatoes, quartered
1/2 sm. onion, sliced
1/2 green pepper, seeded, sliced
1/2 cucumber, sliced
4 sprigs parsley
1 clove garlic
1 tsp. instant beef bouillon
1 tsp. salt (opt.)
1/4 tsp. pepper
2 tbsp. canola (Puritan) oil
2 tbsp. vinegar
3/4 c. cold water
2 ice cubes

Put all ingredients in blender. Cover. Blend 15 seconds or until all ingredients pass through blades. Do not over blend. Serve garnished with toasted croutons, or any of the vegetables used in the soup, thinly sliced or chopped. Makes six servings. Serve cold.

BROWNIES

1/2 c. (1 stick) margarine
1 1/2 (1 oz.) squares unsweetened chocolate
1 c. sugar
2 eggs
1 tsp. vanilla

3/4 c. flour
1/2 tsp. baking powder
1/2 tsp. salt
1/2 c. chopped nuts

Melt margarine and chocolate in saucepan over very low heat. Remove from heat, blend and stir in sugar. Add eggs, one at a time, beating well. Add vanilla. Sift flour, baking powder and salt together and beat into chocolate mixture. Pour into a greased 9" square pan. Sprinkle nuts over top. Bake at 350 degrees for 25 minutes. Cut into squares before completely cooled. *Tip cutting with a plastic knife will make for smoother cutting.

HEARTY ZUCCHINI SOUP

2-4 tbsp. butter or margarine
2 sm. white onions, thinly sliced
1 lg. celery rib, scraped & thinly sliced
1 lg. carrot, scraped & thinly sliced
3 c. chicken broth*
3 med. zucchini, unpeeled & cut into quarters lengthwise & thinly sliced
Salt (opt.) & pepper (to taste)

 *May be made with low salt chicken bouillon granules. In heavy soup pot melt butter or margarine and saute onions, celery and carrot until soft. Stir in 1/2 cup broth and zucchini. Cook until zucchini is tender, 10 to 12 minutes. Add remaining broth and simmer slowly until vegetables are tender, but still hold their shapes. Season to taste. Serve hot, sprinkled with cheese if desired. Serves 6. (May add more carrots and celery if desired.)

PETER'S GRILL VEGETABLE SOUP

1/2 c. onions, 1/2" cubes
1/2 c. celery, 1/2" cubes
1/2 c. carrots, 1/2" cubes
1/2 c. potatoes, 1/2" cubes
1 (16 oz.) can whole tomatoes
1/2 tsp. sugar

1 c. frozen mixed vegetables
5 c. water
Salt & pepper to taste

In a kettle saute onions, celery, carrots and potatoes for about 15 minutes. Add tomatoes, sugar, frozen mixed vegetables and water. Simmer until vegetables are done, about 15 to 20 minutes. Salt and pepper to taste. 6 servings.

TURKEY - STUFFING LOAF

4 tsp. margarine
2 sm. apples, pared & diced
1/2 c. each shredded carrot, diced onion, celery, green bell pepper
13 oz. ground turkey
4 slices bread, cubed
1/2 c. plain low fat yogurt
2 eggs, beaten
1/4 tsp. each poultry seasoning & salt

Preheat oven to 375 degrees. In non-stick skillet, heat margarine until hot. Add apples and vegetables and saute, stirring constantly until apples are soft. Remove from heat and stir in remaining ingredients. Spray a 9 x 5 x 3 inch loaf pan with Pam, transfer turkey mixture to pan. Bake until set, 35-40 minutes. Remove from oven, let stand 5 minutes. Invert on serving plate. Or cook in microwave about 15 minutes. Makes 4 servings. Nutritive Note: Serve size + 1/4 loaf. 330 calories; 33 g. cho; 27 g. pro; 594 mg. sodium; 201 mg. chol.

VEGETARIAN'S SPECIAL K LOAF

5 c. Special K cereal
5 eggs, beaten
1 c. chopped walnuts
1 lg. carton cottage cheese
2 tbsp. McKay chicken seasoning or onion soup mix
1 lg. onion, chopped
Chopped celery, if desired

Saute onion in 1/4 cube margarine. Mix all ingredients together and turn into greased loaf pan. Bake 45 minutes. Freezes well. To serve after freezing, reheat in oven 20 minutes.

POOR MAN'S STEAK - AMISH RECIPE

3 lb. hamburger
1 c. cracker crumbs
Salt & pepper
1/4 c. chopped onion
1-2 cans mushroom soup

Mix well and press onto cookie sheet. Chill overnight to set. Cut in squares, roll in flour and brown both sides. Place in baking dish. Pour soup over meat mixture. Bake at 350 degrees for 1 hour.

OVERNIGHT TUNA CASSEROLE (MICROWAVE)

1 can cream of celery soup
1 c. milk
1 can (6 1/2 oz.) can water packed tuna, drained & flaked
1 c. uncooked elbow macaroni
1 c. frozen peas
1/2 c. chopped onion
1 c. grated Cheddar cheese (reserve 1/4 c.)

Whisk soup and milk in 2 quart microwave safe bowl until blended. Add remaining ingredients except 1/4 cup cheese. Cover and refrigerate overnight. Cover with lid or vented plastic wrap. Microwave on high 15-17 minutes until bubbly. Sprinkle with 1/4 cup cheese. Let stand 5 minutes until cheese melts.

BEEF AND CABBAGE ROLL

1 lb. hamburger, sauteed
1 onion, chopped, sauteed
1/2 head cabbage, sauteed

Add Dijon mustard
Salt & pepper

Roll 2 Pepperidge Farm shells (in freezer section of grocery store) to 4 x 18 inch. Add hamburger mix over roll. Bake at 400 degrees for 20 minutes. Bake at 350 degrees for 20 minutes. Can serve with mushroom sauce or gravy over top.

LOW - CALORIE COOKED DRESSING

1/3 c. instant non-fat dry milk
1 1/4 tsp. dry mustard
1 tsp. salt
1/8 tsp. freshly ground pepper
1 tbsp. all-purpose flour
1 med. egg
1 c. water
2 tbsp. white vinegar
1 tbsp. margarine
Sugar substitute 6 tsp. sugar

Combine dry ingredients in top of double boiler. Beat egg slightly and combine with water and vinegar. Add to dry ingredients slowly, stirring to blend well. Cook over simmering water, stirring constantly until thick and smooth. Remove from heat; add margarine and sweetener, blend well. Pour into 1 pint jar, cover. Store in refrigerator. *Nutrition Note: Up to 1 1/2 tablespoons may be considered free in diabetic exchange. 1 1/2 tablespoons = 21 calories.*

BUTTERMILK DRESSING

1/3 c. low fat yogurt
1/2 c. buttermilk
3 tbsp. reduced calorie mayonnaise
1 tbsp. dry Ranch style dressing mix Combine, cover tightly, keep 5 days. Makes 1 cup. 1 serving = 2 tablespoons. 1 serving = 1/2 fat.

LOW CAL SALAD DRESSING

Mix together and chill: 6 tbsp. lemon juice or vinegar 3 tbsp. onion, finely chopped Dash pepper   Chopped parsley or green pepper, horseradish or mustard may be added if desirable. 1 tablespoon = 3 calories.

DATE DIET SALAD

1 c. pineapple juice
3 tbsp. Sugar Twin
1 env. unflavored gelatin
1 #2 can crushed pineapple, drained
5 tbsp. lemon juice
1/2 c. chopped nuts
1 (3 oz.) pkg. cream cheese
1 tbsp. grated lemon peel
1 c. dates, chopped
Dash of salt

Part 1: Soften gelatin in 1/2 cup pineapple juice; dissolve over hot water. Mix with remaining juice, crushed pineapple and sugar twin. Spray 1 quart mold with Pam, arrange few pieces of dates in bottom. Cover with 1 cup of pineapple mixture. Chill until set. *Part 2:* Blend grated lemon peel, salt and cream cheese. Gradually add the remaining pineapple. Stir in dates and nuts. Pour over first layer in mold and chill until firm.

OAT BRAN MUFFINS

2 1/4 c. oatbran cereal, uncooked
1/4 c. chopped nuts
1/4 c. raisins
2 tsp. baking powder
1/2 tsp. salt
3/4 c. milk
1/3 c. honey
2 eggs, beaten
2 tbsp. vegetable oil

Preheat oven to 425 degrees. Spray 12 medium sized muffin tins with Pam or line with paper baking cups. In large bowl combine oat bran cereal, nuts, raisins, baking powder and salt. Add remaining ingredients; mix just until all dry ingredients are moistened. Fill prepared muffin cups almost full. Bake 15-17 minutes, or until golden brown. Serve warm. 12 servings, *1 serving = 1 muffin. 45 g. chol; 3 g. pro; 5 g. fat; 114 cal; 2.6 g. fiber; 188 mg. sodium; 46 mg. chol.*

HOMEMADE GRANOLA

4 c. quick cooking rolled oats
1/2 c. Grape Nuts cereal
Granulated sugar sub. equal to 1/4 c. sugar
1 c. chopped peanuts
1/3 c. oil
1/2 c. wheat germ
1/2 c. raisins

Spread oats on ungreased baking sheet; bake at 350 degrees for 10 minutes. Combine remaining ingredients except wheat germ and raisins. Bake mixture on another baking sheet for 20 minutes at 350 degrees, stirring once to brown evenly. Cool in oven. Stir oats, wheat germ, and raisins into mixture. Refrigerate in jars or plastic containers. Yield: 6 1/2 cups. Serving size = 1/4 cup. *Diabetic exchange/serving: 1 starch, 1 fat. 140 cal; 15 g. cho; 5 g. pro; 7 g. fat; 57 mg. sodium.*

SUGARLESS CAKE WITH PINEAPPLE

1 c. raisins
1/2 c. dates, chopped
1/2 c. crushed pineapple (packed in juice)
1 c. water
1/4 lb. margarine
1 1/2 c. flour
1 tsp. soda
1 tsp. vanilla
2 eggs
1/2 c. chopped nuts

Boil raisins, dates, pineapple and water for 3 minutes. Add margarine and let cool. Beat eggs and vanilla. Add flour sifted with soda. Add cooled fruit mixture and nuts, mixing well. Pour into greased and floured 9 x 13 inch pan. Bake in 350 degree oven approximately 25 minutes, or until a toothpick in center comes out clean. Cool. May frost with 8 ounce cream cheese mixed with 1/4 cup honey.

SUGARLESS APPLE PIE

6 c. red delicious apples, peeled & sliced
1 (6 oz.) can sugarless apple juice
2 tbsp. cornstarch
1/2 tsp. cinnamon
1/4 tsp. nutmeg
Pastry for 2 crust pie

Simmer apples in juice about 5 minutes. Mix cornstarch and spices with a small amount of water. Add to apples, boil until thickened. Line pie plate with favorite pastry. Add apples. Cover with top crust, seal edges. Bake at 400 degrees until crust is browned. Note: Frozen blueberries may be substituted for apples. Omit the spice. Fresh or frozen peaches may be used instead of apples. Add a little nutmeg, but no cinnamon.

LEAN PIE CRUST

1/2 c. flour
1/4 tsp. salt
1/4 tsp. baking powder
1/4 c. diet margarine

Mix flour, salt and baking powder. Add margarine. Cut with pastry blender until mix does not stick to bowl. Shape in ball. Chill for 1 hour. Roll on floured board. Bake at 425 degrees for 12 minutes. Makes 1 crust.

SUGARLESS COOKIES

1 c. Raisins
1 c. Water

¾ c. Shortening
2 Eggs
1 tsp. Vanilla
1 (6 ounce) can frozen sugarless apple juice thawed and diluted to make 1 1/2 cups liq
3 c. Flour
½ tsp. Baking Powder
1 tsp. Soda
1 tsp. Cloves
2 tsps. Cinnamon
pinch of salt
½ c. Chopped Nuts
1 c. Coconut

Simmer raisins with water for 15 minutes. Drain juice and add enough water to measure 3/4 cup. Cream shortening and eggs. Add vanilla sugarless apple juice thawed and diluted to make 1 1/2 cups liquid. Beat well. Sift together flour, baking powder, soda, 1 teaspoon cloves, cinnamon and salt. Add to egg mixture and beat well. Stir in raisins and the 3/4 cup raisin liquid, chopped nuts and coconut. (A little sugar twin may be added also.) Drop rounded tablespoons on a cookie sheet sprayed with Pam. Bake at 350 degrees, for 10-12 minutes. These freeze well.

ORANGE DATE BARS

1 c. chopped dates
1/3 c. sugar
1/3 c. vegetable oil
1/2 c. orange juice
1 c. flour
1 1/2 tsp. baking powder
1 egg
1 tbsp. grated orange rind

Combine dates, sugar, oil and juice in saucepan and cook for 5 minutes to soften dates. Cool. Add remaining ingredients and mix well. Spread into an oiled 8 x 8 inch baking pan. Bake at 350 degrees for 25-30 minutes. Cool before cutting into 36 bars.

SUGARLESS PRUNE CAKE

1 c. raisins
1 c. prunes
1 c. dates, chopped
2 c. water
2 sticks oleo
2 tsp. vanilla
2 c. flour
1 tsp. salt
1 tsp. cinnamon
2 tsp. soda
4 eggs
1 c. chopped nuts

Boil fruits and water 5 minutes. Add oleo, set aside to cool. Beat 4 eggs. Add vanilla, flour sifted with salt, soda and cinnamon, then fruit mixture and nuts. Mix well. Grease and flour a horn pan, pour in batter. Bake at 350 degrees until a toothpick comes clean. Note: May be baked in several small foil loaf pans, cooled and frozen.

FROZEN BANANA

1/2 banana, peeled
2 tbsp. skim milk
1/4 c. Grape Nuts cereal, crushed to crumbs
Dash of ground cinnamon
Dash of ground nutmeg

Insert an ice cream stick deeply into the cut end of the banana. Dip the banana in milk and roll in cereal crumbs and spices. Wrap in plastic and freeze. Yields 1 serving. Calories = 68. Cholesterol = 16 grams. Protein = 1 gram. Fat = 0 grams.

RED, WHITE & BLUE SALAD

2 c. peeled apples
1/2 c. blueberries, unsweetened

1/2 c. strawberries, unsweetened
1/2 c. grapes

Combine all fruit in bowl. Toss lightly and serve. Yields 7 (1/2 cup) servings. *Exchanges: 1 serving = 1 fruit. Calories per serving = 37. Carbohydrate = 10 grams. Protein = trace. Fat = 0.*

PEANUT BUTTER BALLS

1/3 c. peanut butter
1 tsp. vanilla
2/3 c. unsweetened coconut, shredded
1/4 c. chopped nuts
1 tsp. lemon rind
1/2 c. raisins

Mix all ingredients together. Form into bite size balls. Chill until firm. Yields 14 balls. Exchanges*: 1 ball = 1/2 fruit and 1/2 fat. Calories per ball = 88. Carbohydrate = 6 grams. Protein = 2 grams. Fat = 7 grams.*

MEATLOAF

1 1/2 lb. lean ground beef
1 beaten egg
2 tbsp. chopped onions
1 c. allspice
1 c. corn flakes
1/4 c. water
1/2 tsp. sage
1/2 tsp. garlic

Mix egg, water and corn flakes; let set for 10 minutes. Mix with meat and remaining ingredients. Pack into an oiled loaf pan. Bake at 350 degrees for 1 hour. Yields 9 servings. Exchanges: 1 serving = 3 lean meat and 1 fat. Calories per serving = 186. Carbohydrate = 2.6 grams. Fat = 14.8 grams. Protein = 21.4 grams. Sodium = 45 milligrams. Cholesterol = 86 milligrams.

POPCORN TREAT

1 c. plain popped popcorn (unsalted, preferably air popped)
1 c. bite-size shredded wheat biscuits
2 tbsp. raisins
1 tbsp. dry roasted sunflower seeds
1/2 tsp. ground cinnamon

Mix first 4 ingredients. Sprinkle cinnamon over mixture and toss lightly. (Can be made in larger quantities and stored in an airtight container at room temperature.) Makes 2 cups (2 servings). *Calories = 150 per 1 cup serving. Food exchanges: 1 cup serving = 1 1/2 bread, 1/2 fruit and 1/2 fat. Cholesterol = 27 grams. Protein = 3 grams. Fat = 3 grams.*

BANANA - RAISIN COLE SLAW

2 c. shredded cabbage
1/2 med. banana, chopped
4 tbsp. raisins
1 tbsp. mayonnaise
1/4 tsp. liquid sweetener or 1 pkg. Equal

Mix well and chill. Makes 5 servings. *Exchanges: 1 serving = 1 vegetable, 1 fruit and 1/2 fat. Calories = 60 per serving.*

OATMEAL - FRUIT COOKIES

1 c. flour
1 tsp. baking soda
1/2 tsp. cinnamon
1 c. water
1/2 c. raisins
1/2 c. chopped, pitted dates
1/2 c. chopped, peeled apple
1/2 c. oleo or butter
2 eggs, beaten
1 tsp. vanilla
3/4 c. chopped walnuts

Sift or mix together flour, baking soda and cinnamon; set aside. In 2 quart saucepan over medium high heat bring water, dates, apple and raisins to a boil. Reduce heat to low; simmer 3 minutes. Remove from heat. Add oleo; stir until melted. Pour into large bowl; cool slightly. Add beaten eggs and vanilla. Stir in dry ingredients, oats and nuts. Cover and refrigerate overnight. Drop by heaping teaspoonfuls, 2 inches apart, on greased baking sheet. Bake in 350 degree oven for 12 to 14 minutes. Remove from baking sheet. Cool on racks. Store in refrigerator in airtight container. Makes about 40 cookies.

DIET PUMPKIN PUDDING

1 can (16 oz.) pumpkin
2 c. skim milk
2 eggs
1 tsp. cinnamon, or more
Dash of salt (1/8 tsp.)
1 tsp. vanilla
4 to 5 pkg. Equal to taste

Blend all ingredients. Pour into a casserole bowl. Bake at 425 degrees for 15 minutes, then lower the heat to 350 degrees and bake another 40 to 45 minutes.

BROCCOLI & CHEESE POTATOES

2 baked potatoes
2 tsp. margarine
2 tsp. cornstarch
1/2 c. skim milk
1/8 tsp. dry mustard
4 oz. cheddar cheese, grated
2 c. cooked broccoli

Bake potatoes until done. Cook broccoli in salt water until tender. Melt margarine in saucepan. Add cornstarch, milk and dry mustard; cook until thick. Then stir in cheese until it melts. Stir in broccoli. Split potatoes and top with broccoli mixture. 4 servings. *Exchanges: 1 serving = 1 vegetable, 1 high fat meat, 1 1/4 bread and 1/2 fat.*

Calories = 241 per serving. Fat = 11.5 grams. Protein = 12.5 grams. Carbohydrate = 24 grams.

SUGARLESS BANANA BREAD

1 3/4 c. sifted cake flour
2 tsp. baking powder
1/4 tsp. baking soda
1/2 tsp. salt
1/4 c. melted margarine
2 egg, beaten
Liquid sweetener to equal 1/2 c. sugar
1 tsp. vanilla
2 med. sized bananas, mashed

Sift together flour, baking powder, baking soda and salt. Add remaining ingredients except bananas. Stir only until flour mixture is moistened. Fold in mashed bananas. Pour into greased 8 x 4 inch loaf pan. Bake at 350 degrees until top springs back when touched, about an hour. Yields 14 slices. Exchanges: 1 bread and 1/2 fat. Calories = 109. Carbohydrate = 15 grams. Fat = 4 grams. Protein = 2/5 grams. Cholesterol = 39 milligrams.

STRAWBERRY SHAKE

1/2 c. skim milk
1/2 c. plain low-fat yogurt
1/2 c. frozen unsweetened whole strawberries
1/2 tsp. vanilla extract
1 pkg. artificial sweetener (Equal)

Put all ingredients in a blender or food processor. Blend until smooth and serve. Yields 1 (1 1/2 cup) serving. *Calories = 106. Exchanges: 2/3 fruit, 1 milk and 1/2 fat. Cholesterol = 19 grams. Protein = 8 grams. Fat = 2.5 grams.*

CINNAMON TOAST

1 slice high fiber or high protein whole wheat bread
1 tsp. diet margarine
Ground cinnamon
1 pkg. artificial sweetener (Equal)

Toast the bread. Spread on the margarine, and sprinkle on the cinnamon and sweetener. Yields 1 serving. Calories = 115. Exchanges: 1 bread and 1 fat. Cholesterol = 15 grams. Protein = 2 grams. Fat = 5 grams.

BROCCOLI CASSEROLE

1/2 c. cooked broccoli
1/4 c. cooked rice
1/4 c. cream of mushroom soup (prepared with skim milk)
1 oz. Cheez Whiz
2 oz. browned ground chuck
Dash of onion powder

Mix all ingredients together in a small glass casserole dish. Cover with waxed paper. Bake in microwave oven for 4 minutes at full power. OR, bake in an oven at 350 degrees for 25 to 30 minutes. The recipe can be increased easily to four servings for a family. Yields 1 serving. Exchanges: 1 vegetable, 1 bread, 1 fat and 3 lean meat. Calories = 310.

CASSEROLE SAUCE MIX

2 c. non-fat dry milk
3/4 c. cornstarch
1/4 c. instant chicken broth
2 tbsp. dried minced onion
1/2 tsp. pepper

Combine ingredients and store in airtight container. To use as substitute for ONE can condensed soup, mix 1/3 cup of the dry mix with 1 1/4 cup COLD water in saucepan. Cook and stir until thickened. Add 1 tablespoon margarine, if desired. This will add 11.5 grams of fat. For less calories, sodium and fat; Substitute for cream of chicken, celery or mushroom soups in your recipes. The 1/3 cup with 1 1/4 cup water is equal to 1 can of soup, and there are 95 calories, 0.2 grams fat and 710 milligrams sodium. Campbells canned soup has 330 calories, 23.8 grams fat and 2370 milligrams sodium.

BAKED APPLES

6 or 8 apples
1 can diet strawberry pop
Raisins, if desired

Core apples and place in Pyrex baking dish. Stuff cavity with raisins, if so desired. Pour one can diet pop over apples. Bake in moderate oven (350 to 375 degrees) until apples are tender.

VEGETABLE CONFETTI

1 sm. zucchini, shredded
1 sm. yellow squash, shredded
2 carrots, shredded
1 sm. onion, sliced thin
2 tbsp. water
2 tsp. margarine

Combine the zucchini, yellow squash, carrots, onion, and water in a skillet. Cover and cook over medium heat for 4-5 minutes or until vegetables are tender. Add margarine. Saute, uncovered, until all moisture has evaporated. Serve immediately. Makes 2 servings. *Exchanges: 2 vegetable and 1 fat; calories: 94; carbohydrates: 14 gm; protein: 3 gm; fat: 4 gm; sodium: 83 mg.*

SWEET POTATOES A LA ORANGE

2 lb. sweet potatoes, cooked or 2 lb. vacuum packed sweet potatoes
2 tbsp. margarine, melted
1/2 tsp. ground cinnamon
16 dried apricot halves

Fresh orange slices

Arrange the sweet potatoes in a shallow baking dish. Combine the margarine and cinnamon. Pour over the potatoes. Arrange the apricot halves on top. Cover the dish and bake at 425 degrees for about 15 minutes. Add orange slices and serve. 4 servings. *Exchanges: 1 bread, 1 fruit, 1 fat; calories: 185; carbohydrates: 23 gm; protein: 3 gm; fat: 7 gm; sodium: 79 mg.*

COUNTRY STYLE CHILI

1 lb. ground beef
3/4 c. chopped onion
1 (16 oz.) can kidney beans
1 pt. canned tomatoes (2 c.)
1 (8 oz.) can tomato sauce
1 (4 oz.) can mushrooms, stems and pieces
1 1/2 c. frozen mixed vegetables
1 tsp. chili powder
1 tsp. salt
1/4 tsp. paprika
1 1/4 c. cayenne pepper

Brown ground beef with fat; drain. Add kidney beans, canned tomatoes, tomato sauce, salt, chili powder, paprika, and cayenne pepper. Simmer 1/2 hour. While simmering, cook frozen mixed vegetables according to directions. Add mushrooms and cooked vegetables to chili and simmer for an additional 1/2 hour. 6 servings. *Exchanges: 1 starch, 1 bread, 2 lean meat and 2 vegetables; calories: 246; carbohydrates: 24 gm; protein 23 gm; fat 7 gm.*

HOLIDAY PRUNE AND RAISIN ROLL

1 tbsp. quick rising yeast
3 1/2 to 4 c. flour
1/4 c. white Sugar Twin
1/4 c. soft, light margarine or 1/4 c. safflower oil
1/2 tsp. salt
1/2 tsp. pure lemon extract or 1 tsp. grated lemon rind
1 1/4 c. lukewarm water

1/2 c. Egg Beaters or 2 well beaten eggs
Pam (pan-coating) or other non-stick spray

Combine flour, yeast, salt, white Sugar Twin together in a bowl. In another bowl cream margarine, water, lemon extract, and Egg Beaters. Combine contents of both bowls and mix until dough is soft. Place dough in another bowl (spray with Pam). Cover and let rise 15-20 minutes.

Punch down and let dough rise for an additional 15-20 minutes. While dough is rising: 1/2 c. raisins 1/2 tsp. pure lemon extract Brown Sugar Twin to taste 1/4 c. evaporated skim milk   Cook raisins and prunes in a little water until tender.

Place in blender and mix or mash with potato masher. Add brown Sugar Twin and lemon extract. To prepare roll for cooking: Roll out dough, forming a rectangle. Sprinkle with filling and roll up, sealing edges with a little water.

Place roll on baking sheet, lightly sprayed with Pam. Shape roll into circle or horse shoe. Brush top of roll with evaporated skim milk. Slit top of roll with sharp scissors until some the filling shows through. Bake at 400 degrees for 20-30 minutes or until brown. 35 servings. *Exchanges: 1 starch/bread, 1/2 fruit; calories: 109; carbohydrates: 21 gm; protein: 2 1/2 gm; fat: 2 gm.*

BEEF STEW

1 lb. lean beef, cubed
2 tbsp. Worcestershire sauce
1/2 tsp. salt
1/4 tsp. oregano
1/8 tsp. allspice
1 beef bouillon cube
2 c. boiling water
1 c. canned tomatoes
4 med. potatoes, cubed
3 med. carrots, sliced
3 sm. onions, quartered
1 (10 oz.) pkg. frozen peas

Marinate beef in Worcestershire sauce for several hours. Brown beef cubes in non-stick skillet. Add salt, oregano, and allspice. Dissolve bouillon cube in boiling water; pour over beef. Add tomatoes and simmer over low heat for 1 1/2 to 2 hours or until meat is tender. Add potatoes, carrots, and onions, continue to cook for 30 minutes. Add peas; cook 15 minutes longer or until meat and vegetables are tender. 6 servings. Amount 1 cup. *Exchanges: 1 bread, 2 medium-fat meat, 1 vegetable.*

ITALIAN SPAGHETTI

1/2 sm. onion, chopped
1/2 lb. lean ground beef
1/3 c. tomato paste
2/3 c. water
2 1/4 tsp. Italian seasoning
1/2 tsp. onion powder
1/4 tsp. garlic powder
1/4 tsp. oregano
1/8 tsp. pepper
1 sm. bay leaf
1/2 c. tomatoes, fresh or canned
2 c. cooked spaghetti, drained

Combine onion and ground beef. Place in non-stick skillet and brown, draining off fat as it accumulates. Add tomato paste, water, spices, herbs, and tomatoes. Simmer 1 or more hours, adding more water if needed. Serve 1/2 cup sauce over 1/2 cup cooked spaghetti. 4 servings. *Exchange: 1 bread, 1 vegetable, 1 medium-fat meat.*

SHRIMP SCAMPI

1/2 c. reconstituted dry butter substitute
1/2 tsp. salt
1/2 tsp. garlic powder
1/2 tsp. parsley
1/4 tsp. oregano
1/4 tsp. sweet basil
1/8 tsp. cayenne pepper
1 1/2 c. fat free chicken broth

1 1/2 tbsp. lemon juice
2 c. cooked shrimp, peeled and deveined
1 tbsp. cornstarch

Combine all ingredients except shrimp and cornstarch. Bring to a boil and add shrimp. Stir in cornstarch to thicken. NOTE: Serve over rice or noodles (count as bread exchange). 10 servings. Amount 2 ounces. *Exchange: 2 low-fat meat, 1 vegetable.*

TUNA SALAD

1 (6 1/2 oz.) can water packed tuna
2 hard cooked eggs, chopped
1/4 c. chopped celery
2 tbsp. reduced calorie mayonnaise
Lettuce leaves; optional

Combine all ingredients except lettuce leaves. Refrigerate until served. Serve on lettuce leaf, if desired. 4 servings. Amount 1/2 cup. Exchange: 2 low-fat meat.

DEVILED EGGS

4 hard cooked eggs
1/2 tsp. dry mustard
1/4 tsp. salt
Dash of onion powder
Dash of pepper
2 tsp. reduced calorie mayonnaise
1 tsp. vinegar
Paprika

Halve eggs; remove yolks and mash. Add other ingredients except paprika to mashed yolks; beat well. Refill egg whites with yolk mixture. Sprinkle with paprika. Refrigerate until served. Yields 4 servings. Amount 2 egg halves. Exchange: 1 medium-fat meat.

MACARONI AND CHEESE

1 1/2 c. skim milk
1 1/2 tbsp. all purpose flour
1 1/2 tbsp. reduce calorie margarine
1/2 tsp. salt
3/4 c. grated low-fat American cheese
2 c. macaroni, cooked and drained
1/4 c. bread crumbs

Combine milk, flour, margarine, and salt to make a white sauce. Return sauce to low heat. Add grated cheese, stirring constantly. Cook until cheese has melted and sauce boils. Remove from heat. Alternate layers of macaroni and cheese sauce in non-stick baking dish; cover with bread crumbs. Bake at 375 degrees until mixture bubble and crumbs brown. 6 servings. Amount 1/2 cup. Exchange: 1 bread, 1 medium-fat meat.

DEEP DISH APPLE PIE

Sugar substitute to equal 1/3 c. sugar
1 tbsp. cornstarch
1/2 tsp. grated lemon rind
2 1/2 tsp. lemon juice
1/4 tsp. nutmeg
1/2 tsp. cinnamon
4 sm. apples, sliced
1 c. all purpose flour, sifted
1 tsp. salt
1/4 c. reduced calorie margarine
3 tbsp. cold water

Combine sugar substitute, cornstarch, lemon rind, lemon juice, nutmeg, cinnamon, and apple slices. Place in 9 inch deep dish pie plate on baking dish; set aside. Combine flour and salt; cut in margarine until mixture resembles cornmeal. Blend in water with fork until all dry ingredients are moistened. Shape dough into a ball. Roll out dough on floured surface, and place on top of apple filling. Bake at 425 degrees for 35 minutes or until brown. Cut in 8 equal slices and serve. Yields 8 servings. Amount 1/8 of pie. Exchange: 1 1/2 bread, 1/2 fat.

OATMEAL COOKIES

1 1/2 c. all purpose flour
1 1/2 c. reg. oatmeal, uncooked
Sugar substitute to equal 1/2 c. sugar
1/2 tsp. baking soda
1/4 tsp. salt
3/4 c. reduced calories margarine, softened
3 tbsp. cold water

Combine all ingredients except margarine and water. Cut margarine into dry mixture with pastry blender or knife; blend until mixture resembles coarse meal. Sprinkle cold water over surface; stir with fork until moistened. Roll dough to 1/4 inch thickness on waxed paper. Cut into 24 round or squares. Place cookies on non-stick cookie sheet. Bake at 350 degrees for 15 minutes. Yields 24 cookies. Amount 1 cookie. Exchange: 1 bread.

APPLE CINNAMON OATMEAL

1 1/2 c. water
1/4 tsp. salt
2/3 c. quick cooking oatmeal
1 med. apple, peeled and grated
1 tsp. cinnamon
2 tbsp. raisins
Sugar substitute to taste

Bring water and salt to boil in saucepan. Stir in oatmeal, apple, cinnamon and raisins. Reduce heat and cook 1 minutes until water is absorbed. Serve hot with sugar substitute. Yields 3 servings. Amount 1/2 cup. Exchange: 1 bread and 1 fruit.

BERRY PUDDING

3 c. fresh or frozen unsweetened berries
3 tbsp. cornstarch
1/8 tsp. salt
1/8 tsp. cinnamon
1 c. water

1/2 tsp. vanilla or almond extract
Sugar substitute to equal 1 c. sugar

Combine 1 cup berries, cornstarch, salt, cinnamon, and water in saucepan. Cook over medium heat until mixture thickens, stirring constantly. Add vanilla or almond extract, remaining 2 cups berries, and sugar substitute; mix well. Cool and serve. 6 servings. Amount 1/2 cup. Exchange: 1 fruit.

BISCUITS

1 pkg. dry yeast
2 tbsp. warm water (105-115 degrees)
2 c. buttermilk
5 c. all purpose flour
Sugar substitute to equal 1/4 c. sugar
1 tbsp. baking powder
1 tsp. soda
1 tsp. salt
1 c. shortening

Combine yeast and water; let stand 5 minutes or until bubbly. Add buttermilk to yeast mixture and set aside. Combine dry ingredients in large bowl; cut in shortening until mixture resembles coarse crumbs. Add buttermilk mixture to dry mixture, stirring with fork until dry ingredients are moistened. Turn dough out on floured surface and knead lightly about 3-4 times. Roll dough to 1/2 inch thickness; cut into 36 rounds with a 2 inch cutter and place on non- stick baking sheets. Bake at 400 degrees for 10-12 minutes. Makes 36 biscuits. Serving 1 biscuit. Exchange: 1 bread and 1 fat.

CORNBREAD DRESSING

3 c. crumbled cornbread
1 c. bread crumbs
2 c. fat free chicken broth
1 c. celery, finely chopped
3/4 c. onion, finely chopped
2 egg whites
1/2 tsp. salt

1/2 tsp. pepper
1/2 tsp. poultry seasoning

Combine all ingredients in mixing bowl; mix well. Turn into non-stick dish. bake at 350 degrees for 45 minutes or until light brown and "set". 8 servings. Each serving 3/4 cup. *Exchange: 1 bread and 1/2 fat.*

CREAMED POTATO SOUP

4 med. potatoes, peeled and cut into eighths
1 sm. onion, cut into eighths
4 green onions, coarsely chopped
1 clove garlic, minced
2 (10 1/2 oz.) cans no-salt added chicken broth, undiluted
1 c. skim milk
1/2 tsp. salt
1/2 tsp. white pepper
1/8 tsp. nutmeg

Combine potatoes, onion, green onions, garlic, and broth in a heavy 3 quart saucepan. Cover and simmer 20 minutes or until potatoes are tender. Process potato mixture in batches in container of an electric blender or food processor until smooth. Combine pureed mixture with milk and remaining ingredients, stirring until well blended. Reheat soup to serving temperature or cover and refrigerate until chilled. Amount 3/4 cup. *Exchange: 1 starch, 85 calories.*

CPSIA information can be obtained
at www.ICGtesting.com
Printed in the USA
LVHW060723150621
690190LV00013B/960